COME,
LET US
PLAY
GOD

COME,

✹

LET US

✹

PLAY

✹

GOD

LEROY AUGENSTEIN

1817

HARPER & ROW, PUBLISHERS

NEW YORK, HAGERSTOWN, SAN FRANCISCO, LONDON

First Harper & Row paperback edition published in 1976.

LIBRARY OF CONGRESS CATALOG CARD NUMBER: 68-29567

ISBN: 0-06-060396-8

75 76 77 78 79 10 9 8 7 6 5 4 3 2 1

✖

CONTENTS

PREFACE   vii

1   SHALL WE PLAY GOD?   I

2   AM I MY FETUS'S KEEPER?   16
        Genetic defects

3   CANCEL MY RESERVATION, ST. PETER, I'VE
    DECIDED TO STAY ON!   37
        Organ transplant and death

4   OUR EXPLODING CHALLENGE   54
        Reasons and effects of population explosion

5   THE MONKEY ON OUR BACKS   64
        Responsible population control

6   THE LAST SANCTUARY   80
        Mind and behavior manipulation

7   BUTTON, BUTTON, WHO HAS THE BUTTON?   99
        Who should make decisions

8   ROAD MAP FOR THE UNKNOWN   115
        Abortion legislation as a model

CONTENTS

9   THE HIGH COST OF LIVING   126
      Values for tomorrow's decisions

10 THE DAYS OF OUR ADOLESCENCE   143

    A COMPILATION OF CRITICAL QUESTIONS
      FOR DISCUSSION   147

✖

PREFACE

As the Science Co-ordinator for the Seattle World's Fair in 1961 it was my responsibility to represent all of science. To do this five areas or buildings were established. The first dealt with the history of science; the second with the tools and concepts of science; the third was a science-fiction type treatment of what might be possible in the future; the fourth very large area dealt with research methods and findings; and the final set of exhibits was supposed to treat the impact of science on society. The first four areas almost seemed to develop themselves, but unfortunately the fifth area never jelled. Neither I nor the consultants who worked with me fully saw through the implications of what science is doing to man's concept of himself. That is what this book is all about.

In it I attempt to do three things. First, to bring you up to date in a number of areas of science which I find terribly exciting and important and to anticipate the direction research is likely to go, or even must go. Second, to define the overall ethical dilemmas we face and describe in detail the problems unique to individual developments. Finally, I wrestle with the crucial issue of who should be making these decisions and what values we should use.

Throughout I have followed the somewhat unusual approach of speaking directly to you because the kind of decisions I describe are very personal and usually need to be answered by one or two individuals talking things over.

The actual contents of this book really began to take shape back in 1963. As the chairman of the brand new Department of Biophysics I was asked late in 1962 to appear before the Board of Trustees of Michigan State University and explain what we were planning to do. Many of our plans and hopes were directed at eventually understanding how the mind works. As I talked about our research plans in this area, one of the Board members asked if we were discussing the implications of this with the general public. My answer was no, that I didn't have any opportunities. I was then assured that I would have in the future.

In February of 1963 our provost half asked and half told me to describe some of our research work to a large group of school board members and administrators. He stressed that I should talk at length about the moral and ethical implications of this type of research. I did this reluctantly, because I have no formal training in the humanities at all. To my great surprise, I began to get request after request to speak in this area simply because few other people were willing to speak out about such obviously tricky topics.

Following my early speeches, members of the audiences made the point over and over again that the moral and ethical decisions I was discussing are not unique to mind manipulation—the same questions must be faced in the areas of gene manipulation and birth defects, in the whole area of spare parts, in population explosion, etc.

Further, it became evident as I delved into these areas where I had little formal experience that they were not only the same questions, but that this was what we had missed in designing the final section of the Seattle exhibit on the impact of science on society.

When I early began to comprehend that resolving the critical questions involved really meant making God-like decisions, I almost stopped speaking because I was pessimistic as to whether you the public would be willing to wade through all of the essential scientific details and then face up to the profound and age-old questions involved. Fortunately, I was wrong! After well over 1,000 speeches I now know that you are concerned, you are astute, and you are willing and eager to address yourself to these questions no matter what your age or station in life.

This book is dedicated to you—the public. It is you who have educated me in the subtleties of the problems involved, and I hope that since you have frustrated me with some of your questions, you will in turn be frustrated by many of mine. But above all, I hope you have my sense of urgency. We have 10 to 25 years —at most 50—to set up new decision-making apparatus and answer some profound questions which previously we have left to God.

In recognizing this awesome responsibility, we dare not ever become arrogant or callous, for even though we have no choice but to play a superhuman kind of role, we can never *be* God. However, God has given us dominion over the earth. Since man's increasing knowledge now forces him to make decisions of life and death that cannot be sidestepped, come let us make them together—humbly and prayerfully, but above all responsibly.

LEROY AUGENSTEIN

There is a tide in the affairs of men,
Which, taken at the flood, leads on to fortune;
Omitted, all the voyage of their life
Is bound in shallows and in miseries.
        —SHAKESPEARE, *Julius Caesar*, ACT IV, sc. 3

✳

CHAPTER I

Shall We Play God?*

"Doctor, I realize that I'm asking you to play God, but we need your advice very much. As you know, my grandfather will die in a very short time if he doesn't get a kidney, and all the medical tests indicate that if I donate one of mine he will almost certainly live for a year or more. If I don't do what I can to save his life, I'll never forgive myself. Yet if I do give up one of my kidneys I may be cheating myself and my own family, because then there's a good chance I'll die at a much earlier age than normal. What should I do?"

KIDNEY TRANSPLANT OPERATIONS CAN INDEED LEAD TO TRICKY DECISIONS, I discovered when I was asked by the Chairman of Medical Ethics in another state to give advice on this case. The family involved found themselves in the following circumstance. The sixty-six-year-old grandfather had both kidneys go bad, and there was great difficulty in maintaining adequate function on a kidney machine. When cell matchings were run on the other mem-

*This topic was first given as a lecture in February 1963 before a luncheon of the Michigan Association of School Boards and School Administrators. Portions of this material have been published in *The Centennial Review* for 1964, p. 221; *American Cooperation*, p. 125 (Q1964); and *Christian Century*, October 1967.

bers of the family, it was found that the twenty-two-year-old grandson's cells were remarkably similar to the grandfather's. Thus, if an operation were run, there was a good chance the grandfather would live at least another year and perhaps two or three—at most five more years. However, the loss of one kidney would probably reduce the life expectancy for the grandson by as much as ten years, unless there are some really significant technological developments in the immediate future. In most cases a person with only one kidney has an almost normal life expectancy, but the attending physician said that this was probably not the case here because the grandfather's kidney failure appeared to be the result of a genetic defect that runs in the family.

When I first talked to them the grandson said he was very eager to donate his kidney, whereas the grandfather was dubious as to whether he ought to accept it. Would you recommend to this family that they go ahead with the operation?

Before asking my next question, let me add another piece of information. One reason I was called is that the grandfather was an outstanding surgeon who saves between a hundred and three hundred lives a year. Further, he was still operating, one year past the normal retirement age, because he serves a large, remote area, and for five years they have been unsuccessful in getting a younger man to come in and take over his practice. Now, would you advise the grandfather to accept that kidney? If you are inclined to say yes, do you want to change your vote when I tell you that the grandson has a two-year-old daughter and that his wife is pregnant again? Further, he is a promising graduate student training for medical research. Thus, he might conceivably make some discovery that would save many thousands of lives. However, that is only a hope, whereas the grandfather's ability to save lives is more of a reality even at his advanced age.

With all the facts on the table now, how would you advise this family? Incidentally, would your vote be different if you knew that either the surgeon or his grandson is a nice guy or a foul-tempered so-and-so?

I assume that many people might be uncertain of their decision for the same reasons that I myself vacillated as I learned the facts. I do not feel that it is proper for a person, under any but the most unusual circumstances, to extend his life expectancy by a small degree at the expense of a large chunk of another's life-span. However, how shall one balance the obligations of a father to the young children he has conceived against his responsibilities to unknown strangers whose lives may be lost for lack of a surgeon? Resolving this dilemma requires facing up carefully to two age-old questions: *What is man?* and *Why are we here?*

In the face of this kind of problem, it is unfortunate that ever since Sputnik the myth has grown that if we just have enough research and get enough facts out to the public, somehow everything will come out OK. The above situation clearly illustrates that nothing could be further from the truth.

SCIENCE MARCHES ON, FAST AND FURIOUSLY, BUT ALL TOO OFTEN OUR ABILITY TO HANDLE OUR NEWFOUND POWERS DOES NOT KEEP PACE. Increasingly, the advances being made in many areas of science and technology pose ethical and moral dilemmas which *cannot* be resolved by facts alone. Rather, the proper utilization of our new scientific findings requires that we face up to some terribly critical decisions, based upon our most fundamental values and beliefs.

It cannot be emphasized enough that, as the pace quickens, the gap between our ability to discover and our ability to handle our discoveries becomes ever greater in both magnitude and peril. In the matter of organ transplants, as in many other areas of science, our knowledge is doubling every 7 to 10 years. Yet in putting that knowledge to use we often rely exclusively on beliefs and practices which originated centuries ago, and seem to think that we can take centuries more to reevaluate and perhaps change our operating procedures.

Actually, many of those old beliefs are still valid and should not be discarded casually. As Winston Churchill said, "If we open a quarrel between the past and the present, we shall find that we have lost the future." Yet, by the same token, we dare not refuse to reexamine and reject old comfortable dogmas which are hopelessly oversimplified and no longer pertinent. To do so would be to bury our heads so deeply in the sand that we would surely suffocate. Thus, we have before us a lot of fundamental decisions which should have been made yesterday and cannot wait until the day after tomorrow. Certainly the "two cultures" of C. P. Snow—and particularly science and religion—must beat their swords into plowshares and work together closely and harmoniously.

OUR KNOWLEDGE OF HOW HUMAN HEREDITY IS DETERMINED AND HOW IT MAY BE CONTROLLED IN THE FUTURE HAS RECENTLY BEEN GROWING BY LEAPS AND BOUNDS. Although bits and pieces of this information are announced regularly in the news media, many people are unaware of either the full scope of the discoveries in this area or the capabilities which this new information provides us—or, most importantly, the ethical implications. One case may serve to provide a partial assessment of our new powers and their ramifications.

Recently a very fine Jewish couple came to my office seeking scientific advice. Thirteen years prior to their visit, there was born to them a beautiful little girl, who developed brilliantly, was well adjusted socially—all in all, it was one of those absolutely delightful family situations. Tragically, when the child was eight years old and began to have trouble in seeing, their doctor gave them the dread diagnosis: she had amaurotic idiocy. This meant that the insulation —the myelin sheath—surrounding the optic nerve had begun to develop abnormal fatty deposits, so that the optic nerve no longer functioned properly. Unfortunately, the degeneration proceeded on back into the central nervous system, with the result that the child began to have seizures and convulsions, and over a six- to eight-month period died a brutal death. Although they had taken strong contraceptive measures against having further children, they were now in my office because the mother had accidentally become pregnant once more.

They immediately asked, "What are the chances for a repeat on this new pregnancy?" The answer: 25 per cent! because amaurotic idiocy is a recessive trait which will not appear unless we get a gene of a particular kind from each parent. Since neither parent had the failing, obviously neither of them had two defective genes; yet each had contributed one to the child, and thus we knew that each parent had one good and one defective gene for this trait. Thus, in any procreation in which these two were involved, the chances would be one out of four that the two defective genes would again combine and the cycle repeat itself.

They immediately asked if I were absolutely sure that they were each carrying the defective gene. I had to answer, "Pretty sure, but not absolutely." My slight uncertainty arose as follows. Although amaurotic idiocy is very prevalent in the Jewish community (some estimate that 1-2 per cent of those of Jewish descent in the New York area carry a defective gene for this trait), their children normally die in the first year of life. It is in another north European variation that the child normally lives to an age somewhere between seven and twelve. A later check of the family tree of this couple showed that they had had a common Scottish ancestor, four generations back on one side and five on the other: presumably this was the source from which this particular gene had come into their genetic pool.

It is now possible to run a test to determine, with some degree of accuracy, whether an individual is a carrier of a good and a bad gene in this respect. Blood cells are taken from the patient and stained with either of two dyes. Many times, in people who are carriers, 1.5 per cent of the cells already show the abnormal fatty deposit: apparently with one good and one bad gene there is some degeneration, but it does not get out of hand. Although they were warned that these tests do not always give a definite answer, these parents requested that arrangements be made for the testing and the laboratory results indicated that both parents were almost certainly carriers.

Their final question was as follows. "All right our chances are one out of four that the child will again be defective, but they are three out of four that it will be normal. Can you give us any information at all about whether we have hit the one out of four or the three out of four possibility with this particular fetus?" Since there was a long-shot chance that it might be possible to give them an answer, arrangements were made through their family physician to take some cells from the fluid in the amniotic sac surrounding the child in the mother's womb. These cells were sent off to a laboratory along with the blood cells from the parents and were stained in the same way.

Three weeks later their doctor told them that whereas 1.5 per cent of their own cells showed the abnormal fatty deposits, 3.4 per cent of the cells from the fetus had shown this degeneration. Neither the physician nor I knew of comparable tests on cells taken from any other mother's womb during pregnancy, although tests have been run for other suspected defects as we shall see in the next chapter. Even so, on the basis of this information, it seemed fairly likely that this child again had two defective genes.

About a week later the couple asked if they might now talk to me, not about science, but about what I would do if I were in their position. I explained that I could not really put myself in their shoes, for as a practicing Protestant I believe that a fetus is a life, whereas on the basis of their liberal Jewish tradition they felt that life only begins at the time of birth. Within this restriction, I tried to point out to them the pros and cons of whatever action they might take. For example, I emphasized that if the tests were misleading and the child born were actually normal, it would certainly be a blessing to everyone concerned, since it would find itself in the home of two fine human beings who had already given much to society, and who very much wanted a child. Accordingly, I urged them to consider whether they could steel themselves to the possibility that the child might again begin to degenerate after a few years of life. The mother immediately responded, "But don't you realize that we won't be able to get a good night's sleep until that child is at least fifteen years old and we know it's safely past the danger point?" She was right—that is an awfully long stretch of insomnia! Moreover, since the mother was a very concerned and sensitive human being, I knew that she would almost certainly "come apart at the seams" if this child, too, began to show the signs of amaurotic idiocy. In fact, probably few people could survive such an ordeal twice in a lifetime.

What would you advise these people, if they asked you whether they should or should not have an abortion? Clearly, anyone who addresses himself responsibly to this question must consider very carefully what might be the role of this child if it were to come into the world. Once again, we are back to the two questions: *What is man?* and *Why are we here?*

But let me go on and discuss still another area of science before returning again to these two questions, which, even though they are age-old, are becoming ever more critical and pertinent.

HOW THE MIND FUNCTIONS IS ONE OF THE MOST EXCITING, FRUS-TRATING, AND EXPLOSIVE AREAS OF RESEARCH TODAY. Within this vast subject, one of the really fascinating questions pursued by many researchers is, "What kinds of chemical changes correspond to learning?" Although most of us doing research on the mind are interested ultimately in understanding the chemistry of thinking, learning, and memory in man, some of the most tantalizing and controversial experiments with a bearing on the subject have been done with primitive organisms such as the flatworm Planaria. At first glance this might seem like an unusual creature to work with, since it hardly has even what we would normally refer to as a central nervous system. Nevertheless, it has two important properties which have made it valuable for research.

First, in spite of their meager brain apparatus, these little beasts can be taught to do at least eight or nine simple tricks! For example, if you pass a current of electricity through a trough in which they are swimming, they will hunch up and throw their heads to one side in a very characteristic gesture. On the other hand, if you shine a light of moderate intensity on them they will normally pay little attention, even though they have rudimentary eyes. Thus, if you shine a light for exactly three seconds, and shock them during the last half-second only, initially they only hunch up when the shock comes and pay no attentionto the light. However, if the light and shock are presented repeatedly in this fashion, after a hundred times they begin to recoil when the light comes on without waiting for the shock. In fact, after about 300 to 500 trials, they hunch up 90 per cent or more of the time when the light first comes on. In this sense they have been trained as Pavlov trained his dogs. The light to which the Planaria previously paid little attention now signals the onset of something to which they must react.

The ability to learn simple reactions like this however, is not enough to make these animals valuable research tools. They assume experimental importance only when this capability is coupled with a second property. If you cut them in two, the front end grows a new behind while the back end grows a new head. Accordingly, we can use these animals to investigate a question which must be important, since my sergeant in the Army asked it so often: "Are your brains in your head or in your behind?" Actually, they are in both ends of the worm about equally. This conclusion comes from the following experiment. If you train a group of them to recoil at least 90 per cent of the time when the light first comes on, then cut them in two, set them aside until they regenerate the appropriate end, and retrain them, you find interestingly enough that it requires only half as many trials to get them back up to a 90 per cent response level. Furthermore, this does not mean that we have "cut the knowledge in two" for if control animals are trained but then set aside without cutting on the shelf for the ten to fourteen days normally needed to grow a new end they forget half their learning and also have to be retained back to the 90 per cent response level.

Planaria have another interesting property. If you cut them into small pieces, and throw them into the dish with their previous friends, the latter will ingest the pieces just as readily as they do the morsels of liver they are normally fed. From this observation, my good friend Dr. James McConnell of the University of Michigan has developed a most controversial claim: namely, that if you feed pieces of a well-trained worm to a naïve, untrained animal, it takes less time to train the cannibal. According to recent reports, this is a ansfer of specific learning rather than a general enhancement of the ability to be trained.*

In spite of the excitement and potential impact of learning research, there is other work on how the mind functions which must be of even more immediate concern to us. This has been done at McGill University and is concerned with methods of persuasion. Initially the problem posed was: What happens to an individual placed in isolation? Specifically, what happens when you drastically reduce the input of sensory information? To investigate this, Dr. Hebb and his group paid students a little less than a dollar an hour to see how long they could stay in an isolation room. Many students refused to stay more than a day and some complained bitterly that

---

*Needless to say, these reports concern many of us in education, since this suggests a good use for ground up old professors and schoolteachers. In fact, one clergyman pondered whether it might not be possible to have "instant religion" or, as he called it, "redemption by digestion."

this was worse than Hitler's torture. When the students made repeated attempts to increase communication with those on the outside, the experimenters decided to see, "What will they accept for communication?" Accordingly, they installed a switch so that the students could start a boring recording of stock market quotations, or a lecture on alcoholism prepared for 5th and 6th graders, etc. Practically all of the 70 or so college students who stayed in the room for 3 days or more played these recordings repeatedly. The experimenters then asked themselves, "Are they listening to this junk, or is it just to break the monotony?"

In still other experiments, students heard recordings telling them why they should believe in ghosts, or flying saucers, or the ability of some people to talk to spirits or to communicate with others by extra sensory perception, etc. Students who were not in the isolation room would listen to a recording only once and had no further interest. By contrast two thirds of the students in isolation not only wanted the recordings played again, but showed changes of attitude: afterward, one subject said that for the first time in his life he felt uneasy passing a graveyard, while another reported trying to mentally influence the fall of the cards while dealing. These results suggest that under sensory deprivation apparently a person's mind will erase some information and write in, or at least overwrite, new information. This is further suggested by informal reports of a few attempts to change people's attitudes while they are under the influence of what might be called "isolation drugs" rather than being in an isolation room. The reports from Korea and S. Viet Nam also suggest that some drastic changes can be made in a person's basic beliefs and attitudes.

Clearly, such techniques can be used for fantastic good or fantastic evil. Consider for a moment that 50 per cent of our hospital beds are occupied by mental patients. If only we could develop such methods to retrieve psychotic patients, it would be one of the finest gifts any scientist could give to society. By the same token, we know what the Chinese Communists did with this thing called brainwashing.

Here is the dilemma. Information about how the brain works is neither good nor bad per se. The goodness and badness come when we determine *which individuals or groups are to decide* what is bad and to be erased, and what is good, to be written in new. Quite clearly we cannot really determine "good" and "bad" unless we carefully consider our two persistent questions: What is man? Why is he here?

Although many of the critical decisions about mind manipulation and control of human heredity will be made 10, 25 or 50 years from now, we must reconsider our two underlying questions as we deal *today* with problems such as—who is to get a scarce heart? Who is to have the use of a kidney machine which cannot handle all the people who need treatment? Under what conditions should we release some of the potent new drugs for testing in man? In particular, we should be facing up to these two questions right now because of the most overwhelming problem facing mankind today—the *population explosion*. As will be emphasized in Chapter 5, we must soon say, "That child shall not be conceived so that other children already here can have fruitful lives." In so doing we must consider: What might that child's life have been if it had been born?

Quite clearly scientific advances are generating really tough questions. Yet if you have not thought along these lines before, it may be difficult to grasp immediately how complex they are. Let me tell a story here which may demonstrate the kind of complexity we must face.

DECISIONS ABOUT NUCLEAR TESTING RAISE SIMILARLY COMPLICATED ISSUES. In 1956 Adlai Stevenson proposed, as part of his presidential campaign, that we should unilaterally stop testing bombs. Since I worked at Brookhaven National Laboratory, one of our big nuclear installations, I was asked to participate in a public forum on this question. The first man told how Linus Pauling, an eminent scientist, had calculated that the fallout from each hydrogen bomb tested would produce ten thousand leukemic children. He added that nothing can be worth this, so we must stop testing immediately. Another man jumped up and said, "Just a minute! I've just come back from India, where each year one per cent of the population—that's four million people—die of malnutrition, and the reason is that fifty per cent of their heat, light, and power is obtained by burning dried cow dung. If we could provide them with some cheap source of power, then they could put this manure on the fields and go a long way toward solving their malnutrition problems." Thus, if we could explode a hydrogen bomb and bring hydrogen power one year closer, then perhaps we should place on one side of the scales ten thousand children who die of leukemia and on the other side four million Indians who do not die of malnutrition. Put in this way it would be very cruel, but a black-and-white decision. We are comparing numbers of people who die by two different means.

Let me now emphasize that we know this is a false oversimplified comparison. Unfortunately exploding hydrogen bombs has *not* provided technological breakthroughs which have brought hydrogen power one year closer. The thing it buys, if anything, is political stalemate, and I value this highly since I have been behind the Iron Curtain, and I have had numerous Iron Curtain people working in my lab. By the same token, hydrogen bombs apparently do not produce ten thousand leukemic children. The price doesn't seem to be that high, though it isn't zero. We are going to produce some genetic damage in future generations, and even one defective child is tragic.

Now you see the point I am trying to make. Our cruel but black-and-white comparison has gone out the window. We are no longer comparing numbers of people who die from two different causes. No, the thing we are buying is political stalemate. The price we are paying is genetic damage in future generations. How do you compare the value of two such different commodities? Unfortunately, this is the kind of complexity we will have to face more and more—not less and less. Thus, we must be aware of an important historical point.

IN THE PAST WE HAVE DONE A LOUSY JOB WHENEVER SCIENCE HAS FORCED SOCIETY TO FACE UP TO THESE QUESTIONS—WHAT IS MAN? WHY IS HE HERE? The controversy over nuclear testing is only the most recent of many. One of the first occurred when Copernicus said that the earth is not the center of the universe, but only a speck of dust. People said this was downgrading man and could not be so, and we had a hundred years of controversy. Then along came Darwin and said that man was not created from a ball of clay, but rather evolved through many millions of years. Again people said this was downgrading man and thus could not be so. Hopefully we are at the end of that 125 years of controversy. Quite obviously, science is now generating another controversy, but this time it will be quite different.

Now, instead of downgrading man, science is literally forcing us to play God. And let's make no mistake about it, we do this to a certain extent all the time. Every time you throw a pesticide onto the garden, and the bugs go away and so do the robins, you are playing God. Every time a surgeon picks up a scalpel to correct a defect in a person, he is playing God. Every time a minister tries to manipulate a parishioner's basic concepts, he is playing God. In fact, each of us is here right now because two people played God —they procreated a life; nothing is more sacred than that. Thus this is not something new! The big change is that the ante in this poker game has gone sky-high. Or to put it another way we are suddenly going from the sandlots to the major leagues.

MUST WE PLAY GOD DELIBERATELY AND EXTENSIVELY BY MAK-ING SUCH AWESOME DECISIONS? The answer is a definite yes. In fact, we no longer have any option as to whether we will or will not "play God." Once these new tools become available, no matter what we do we *shall be* playing God. Let me return to the case of the Jewish couple to illustrate why I am so positive on this point.

As far as I am concerned, anyone who votes for an abortion is taking a life. By the same token, anyone who says no to aborting the fetus in question is consigning those parents to endless worry, and almost certainly to a nervous breakdown if the child proves abnormal as suggested by the tests. Further, once the child develops amaurotic idiocy symptoms, that no vote has sentenced him to a long siege of dreadful suffering. Thus, either a yes or no represents a very godlike decision. Moreover, anyone who even becomes involved in counseling in such a situation assumes an awesome responsibility.

This was one of the finest couples I have ever met. The man was an outstanding professional with a solid state-wide and budding national reputation. The mother was a very sensitive, promising young artist. Both were highly intelligent and well educated. Quite obviously they were more than capable of making up their own minds—probably more so than practically anyone who could presume to counsel with them. Accordingly, those of us from whom they sought advice (at least those I knew) were very careful to point out to them the ramifications of the various actions they could take, but none of us, I learned later, ever presumed to give them specific advice about what they should do.

Finally, for better or worse, they decided to have an abortion. Since the mother was now well into the fifth month of the pregnancy, it was necessary to secure the services of a very excellent surgeon. Someone—I don't know who—made arrangements for this to be done in Puerto Rico, and so the mother flew down and checked into one of the luxury hotels. As luck would have it, a very talkative woman in the adjacent room invited herself to dinner. When this neighbor asked why she was there, the Jewish lady said that she needed medical treatment. When the talkative lady found out who her doctor was, she said, "Oh, he aborted me a few days ago," and then gave a fairly brief account of the abortion, with much longer and more lurid details of how she had become pregnant.

From even the brief description given here, it should be obvious that the couple had not made their decision in a casual way, but very deliberately. Nevertheless, the wife decided she wanted no part of this kind of tawdry business and accordingly took the first plane back home. Six days later she miscarried naturally and suddenly decided she had been wrong all along, that her fetus was a life, and that this was the wrath of God descended. She is now committed to a mental institution.

Certainly, those of us who talked to the couple can give reasonable and legitimate arguments that we were right in not assuming the burden of making their decision for them. Yet the fact remains that if I or any of the other three had told them what they should do, probably the outcome would have been different. I certainly knew what they wanted to do: in fact, I probably would have done the same thing in their situation in spite of our differing viewpoints as to whether the fetus is or is not a life. Thus if I had said yes, by all means go ahead and have this abortion, and argued with them as to why, very probably during the critical two or three days this mother could have blamed and cursed this guy Augenstein who had given her bum information. But probably she would be sane today.

We are not God, and can never be, since man is only finite and of himself can never know the absolute truth. But participating in the gathering of this kind of information and in the decision-making itself is nothing less than playing at being God. Thus, again I emphasize that no matter what one might have done in this counseling situation, and no matter what this couple might have done—whether their decision was positive or negative—we played God.

HOW DO WE PROCEED IF THIS IS SO? First, it is important to realize that crucial decisions are being made even now. In 1962 my wife and I moved to Lansing, Michigan and bought a house on an acre of land. The only question asked was whether we had enough money. Yet when the house was built, a decision was made in regard to future population levels, for as long as my house and those trees stand on that acre, it cannot be used to produce food to support more people. Every time a superhighway is built, a decision about future population is made. Did you know that approximately 4-5 per cent of the arable land in this country is now covered by asphalt and concrete? That is an area the size of the state of Georgia. Thus we are making decisions, but unfortunately making them by default.

How, then, ought we to make these decisions? We won't go to the polls some bright November day and vote, "Yes, we are going to play God," or "No, we are not." It is to be hoped that we will sneak up on these questions a little more gradually than that. I, for one, would not want Goldwater and Johnson, or Nixon, Humphrey, and Wallace, to sit down in an hour's television debate—or even in a week's White House Conference—and decide a set of new rules and regulations. We must hope that the impetus for these kinds of decisions will come from people like ourselves: that is, from below and not from above.

Beyond all else, we must have carefully considered decisions which avoid the simplistic temptations of the extremists, because the stakes are so desperately high. One of the symptoms of any decaying society has been that philosophical developments have not gone hand in hand with technological developments. In ancient Greece philosophy got far ahead, and they were destroyed from without. In Rome the opposite was true: technology got miles ahead of philosophical developments, and they decayed from within. Sure, the Huns came along and finished them off, but it was a terribly hollow shell they pushed over. Most of us admire not only the durability of the British Empire, but also the way in which for a few centuries they developed together so wonderfully their political institutions, religion, and science.

Only a blind fool could look at our society today and say that philosophical and technological developments are in harmony. If we continue to have what C. P. Snow has called the separation of the two cultures, then I think that like earlier societies, we shall decay very rapidly. It is only too apparent that decisions in the areas already mentioned, and to be considered further in subsequent chapters, require the participation of the scientist with his knowledge and tools. They also require a consideration of values, and so the humanist must participate. Thus, these two groups of people must never be antagonists, since each contributes something essential and neither group alone can resolve our dilemmas. Further, they must work carefully with the politicians who know how to set up a proper apparatus to make and carry out decisions.

Once we have the significant information, no matter what we do in many of these situations, we must make decisions. Accordingly, the only question is *how* we shall go about it and *how well* we shall prepare ourselves. In particular our youngsters, who themselves will have to take many of these decisive stands, must have the proper background and values. Let us explore further what knowledge we must have and what questions we must face if we are to proceed responsibly.

"Of a truth, men are mystically united:
A mysterious bond of brotherhood makes all men one."
—CARLYLE, *Essays, Goethe's Works*

✤

CHAPTER 2

Am I My Fetus's Keeper?*

A MOTHER: I don't think we should ever do anything to prevent the conception or the birth of a defective child like our Suzy. I believe she is part of God's plan. We never knew what love was all about until she came into this world. In fact; if it weren't for her and others like her, maybe you scientists wouldn't be motivated to discover all of these cures which benefit everyone.

AUGENSTEIN: Let me ask you two questions. Do you really believe that you and your husband can ever justify learning to love, if your child has to pay the price of a lifetime of extreme suffering? And can you believe in a God who would give you your wonderful brain and then not expect you to use it to spare Suzy her continual, aimless misery—if you could? That is not the God I believe in! In fact, I don't need suffering little Suzies to spur me on. Rather I need to be sure that people like you will use new information responsibly and humanely. Otherwise we scientists might as well stop right now.

Even though relatively few people are aware of the extent to

*This general material was presented first in 1965 as a speech to a convention of representatives of the Congregational Churches of Michigan. Portions have been published in the *Journal of Home Economics* for October 1967, and the *Humanist*, November 1968.

which birth defects can be anticipated and in a few cases prevented, I still receive about two hundred letters and phone calls each year from people who either fear they may have a defective child or have already had one. They all want to know, "Where do we go from here?" Two case histories will illustrate what we can and cannot do in this whole area.

About five years ago I heard from a couple who had a daughter of twenty, a son of eighteen, and another son in his teens, and then five years prior to writing their letter, they had had a set of twins who were born with microcephaly. Literally this term means "microscopic head"—actually the twins had heads about two thirds of normal size, so that a number of the vital mental functions simply did not operate. Both were blind; one had been born deaf, and the other had a rare blood disorder which made life terribly unpleasant. Both had epileptic seizures. One twin, moreover, at the age of five years weighed only seventeen pounds. Since she screamed from sixteen to eighteen hours a day, she didn't eat very often.

The question posed by the mother was as follows: "Our daughter is just about to become engaged. What are the chances, if she marries and has children, that this will strike again?" Such a dilemma would be of tremendous concern to any family. It was doubly so here, since they were not only a devout Catholic family but a conservative one, which still adhered strongly to the old beliefs about having children once you are married. I shall return to this letter later since it is extremely difficult to deal with scientifically.

The second letter dealt with a defect which is much easier to diagnose accurately, though equally tragic, since it dealt—alas!—with a child of some quite good friends of mine. This couple wrote that their second baby had been found to have muscular dystrophy. Their question came in two parts: "What are the chances that any future children of ours would be stricken with this crippling condition? And can you tell us whether our supposedly normal first child is in fact carrying the seeds of this defect in a hidden form?"

FOR MANY PARENTS WE CAN NOW PREDICT WITH CONSIDERABLE ACCURACY WHAT THEIR CHANCES ARE TO HAVE A CHILD WITH ANY ONE OF A LARGE NUMBER OF DEFECTS. Thus, we were able to give this couple definite answers to both questions. With only a little additional investigation it was possible to tell that their chance for a repeat of muscular dystrophy in a future child was one out of four. This prediction arises as follows.

We each get half of our hereditary material from each parent. In many cases if we get one gene of a particular kind from either parent—it doesn't matter which one—we will exhibit that particular "dominant" trait. Brown hair and brown eyes fall in this category.

Many other dominant traits are not nearly as pleasant to have. For example, achrondroplasia is one of the more common forms of dwarfism. A person's trunk develops fairly normally, but the legs are quite short and usually deformed. Huntington's chorea is another dominant trait. This is a form of spastic seizure that normally sets on in the twenties and is part of what we call St. Vitus's dance.

The important point is that a person who has any dominant trait will pass it on to his offspring with a 50-50 probability. This is true of all the more than 500 dominant traits which we now consider to be defective.

There are many traits, though, which we call recessive, for which one gene is not enough. It is necessary to get a gene of that particular kind from each parent. The particular form of muscular dystrophy in this child falls in this category, as does the amaurotic idiocy mentioned in Chapter 2. Blond hair and blue eyes also fall in this category. Thus while both my wife and I have brown hair and brownish eyes, our son is sandy-haired and blue-eyed. His recessive genes were carried by my wife and myself in a hidden form from two grandmothers who were both blue-eyed.

We now know of at least 500 different recessive elements we consider defective. Included are traits such as cystic fibrosis, PKU, and others, which will be discussed later.

In the case of my friends, neither had muscular dystrophy, so neither of them had two defective genes. Yet the muscular dystrophy in the second child was of the type that indicated it had gotten a defective gene from each parent, so we immediately knew that each of them had a good and a bad gene for this trait. If this couple had any additional children the chances would be one in four that a given child would have two good genes and have no problems whatsoever; would be 50-50 that the child would have a good and a bad gene and be a carrier, like its parents, but not affected; and finally there would be one chance in four that the child would receive two defective genes and again be a cripple. This one-out-of-four chance for a repeat holds for all recessive traits when the parents are carriers but do not exhibit the trait themselves.

In addition to the above, there is one other type of trait which does not fit neatly into the dominant-recessive classification. Mongolism is caused when a child gets one extra chromosome. Instead of the usual 23 chromosomes from the mother and 23 from the father, this child is unlucky: it gets one extra from its mother—and the extra chromosome is the tiniest of them all. Human chromosomes vary by a factor of about 5 in length and are numbered in sequence accordingly. Number 1 is longest, and 22 is tiniest—the twenty-third pair are the two sex chromosomes. The extra chromosome can come along in two different ways.

In a so-called *translocation* mongoloid the extra one adheres to one of the longer, middlesized chromosomes, so that the child gets two normal No. 22's, while the third comes along stuck to another longer chromosome. For parents who have one such "piggy-back" mongoloid child the chances for a repeat are somewhere between 1 out of 6 and 1 out of 3.

In many cases, however, the child just gets three No. 22 chromosomes floating free. The probability for having one of these so-called *trisomic* mongoloids depends strongly upon the age of the mother, although it also appears that such children are born with increasing frequency after viral infections such as hepatitis. The reported correlation with age is as follows: for a mother of age 15, the chances reported by C. S. Reed in his book *Counseling in Medical Genetics* are 6 out of 10,000; at age 20 they are even lower at 2 out of 10,000. Then they go up rapidly! By age 30 the chances are about 1/1000; at age 40, they are 1/100 and if a woman becomes pregnant between 45 and 49 years her chances are somewhere between 1 in 40 and 1 in 25. These statistics indicate why in the past mongoloids have been called "children of a tired womb." There are 8,000 such youngsters born in the United States each year.

Let me now return to the second question asked by my young

friends. Unfortunately, with recessive traits it is necessary in most cases to wait until the first defective child is born before we know that both parents are carriers of a defective gene. In fact, only in the last few years has there been any hope of searching for recessive genes in a person we suspect of having a good and a bad gene for a particular trait.

THERE ARE CURRENTLY TESTS FOR SEEKING OUT 19 DIFFERENT RECESSIVE GENES IN PARENTS. However, in only 6 or 7 of these do we get a definitive answer close to 100 per cent of the time. In many of the others we get a definite yes or no only about 50 per cent of the time, and for some only 10 per cent of the time.

The test for detecting a recessive gene for muscular dystrophy is quite complicated. It is necessary to take a biopsy (small snip of tissue), usually from the large leg muscle, and grow it until quite a few cells are obtained. These cells are then tested for the biochemical abnormality which causes the muscle cells to turn into fatty tissue. Since it is a fairly tedious and complicated set of tests, a definite yes or no is obtained less than half the time.

We knew that, since the first child was not crippled it had either a good and a bad gene or two good genes. The chance of its being a carrier was actually two out of three. The tests were run, and in this case a fairly clear-cut answer was obtained—the "normal" first child was carrying a recessive gene for muscular dystrophy.

The letter from my friends, like about a third of those I receive, ended with the phrase, "Any help you could give us would be very much appreciated." The ability to predict parents' chances for having a defective child is one type of help. A second kind of help would be to go in and chemically correct the defective gene.

THE CHEMICAL MANIPULATION OF HUMAN GENES IS NOW A DISTINCT POSSIBILITY. Thus, it is important to assess just where we stand in this area.

In 1940 a group won the Nobel Prize for changing the heredity of bacteria. They took bacteria with obvious and known properties, ground them up, and extracted their DNA (our chemical shorthand for deoxyribonucleic acid). This hereditary chemical is the stuff of which genes and chromosomes are made. The DNA taken from these bacteria was then put into a second type of bacteria, which behaved quite differently even though the two strains were related.

Lo and behold, some of the second type were transformed—that is, they began to behave like the first! This is analogous to bringing a new plant manager into our Oldsmobile plant in Lansing, Michigan and discovering after a week that the plant is making Fords or Plymouths. In fact, it is one of those analogies which is unbelievably accurate.

Although for almost thirty years, now, we have been able to transform bacteria, we have not been able to do it in human beings *in a controlled way*. Nevertheless, all of us have had many of our cells transformed by viruses. These submicroscopic particles are really packaged nucleic acid.

Many viruses are shaped like a rod with the protein forming the outer coat and the nucleic acid in the hole in the middle of the pipe. Some of the viruses which cause sore throats are shaped essentially like a diamond with one corner whacked off. One of the most-studied viruses is actually shaped like a lollipop with six threadlike filaments on the handle part which serve to attach the virus to the wall of the cell it is attacking. In the business end of these viruses there is also a special chemical which dissolves a hole in the cell wall, and then the DNA that is coiled up in the head of our lollipop is either injected into the cell or slurped in—we aren't sure which, but the head of the virus is seen to collapse after the DNA has infected the cell.

If one of these little "bundles of joy" comes up to one of our cells, we normally say that we could do without this kind of transformation because we end up with a stuffy nose, fever blister, polio, or leukemia. However, we have known for years that if we could figure out how the DNA does this controlling, then in theory we could make good made-to-order genetic changes.

This now appears to be in fact entirely feasible and controllable for one type of human gene. It came about as follows.

At Oak Ridge National Laboratory in Tennessee a group doing research on a rabbit virus found that when their workers went for their annual physical checkups many of them had an abnormally high level of a biochemical called arginase in their blood stream. The experimenters concluded that the nucleic acid in this virus probably contained the necessary instructions for a cell to make arginase, and their workers had a high level of this material because they had become accidentally infected with the rabbit virus. The possibility is of potentially great importance, since there are quite a few people in this country who cannot make their own arginase and as a consequence have a very severe mental retardation. Thus, it was conjectured that if the virus were injected into these people it might transform them so that they could make their own arginase, and their mental retardation might be repaired.

Putting this into a more familiar perspective, it should be pointed out that if we could find a similar virus with the requisite DNA in it, we should be able to cure diabetes. In that case one shot would presumably put the necessary DNA into the pancreas cells, so that a diabetic could make his own insulin and we would no longer have to give him either pills or shots.

What a wonderful boon it would be for medicine, if we could find the necessary viruses to correct some of the most disastrous defects. A problem arises, though, because in many cases you cannot wait until the child is born, or matures, and asks for the treatment himself. If you wait until a microcephalic child appears with a head which is only two-thirds of the normal size, or a mongoloid who has all the abnormal brain connections, you are too late. In those and many related cases it would be necessary to make the corrections even before conception. At least for the recessive genes this could be done in either the sperm or the egg, since if the child gets a good gene from either parent it will be all right.

The sperm would be a bad place to try it, since there are hundreds of millions to a few billion sperm in an ejaculation, and this is just too large a number to treat effectively. The eggs would seem to be a much better place to work.

If we do want to play this game, then it will be necessary to infect a potential mother with an appropriate virus which will get the necessary DNA into the egg cells in her ovaries. At the time of puberty she has only some 100,000 eggs, and unless she comes from a family in which twins and triplets occur repeatedly, she will probably only ovulate one egg each month. This grand total of 300 to 500 during her reproductive lifetime is a treatable number.

To provide a perspective of just where we stand in our research in this area, it should be pointed out that to accomplish this type of genetic transformation it will be necessary to (1) define what is a "good" gene, carrying the right kind of DNA; (2) isolate that DNA for making the copies needed; (3) make many copies of it; (4) find a virus which is specific for eggs in the ovaries; and then (5) take apart the protein outer coat of the virus, remove the unwanted DNA, and replace it with "good" DNA. At the moment we do not have a virus specific for eggs, but some viruses specific for ovarian tissue are known in laboratory animals and probably such a virus could be isolated with five to ten years of very hard work by two or three outstanding labs. At least one—a plant, not an animal, virus—can be disassembled and its nucleic acid removed and replaced, so that presumably once a virus specific for eggs is found, the dissassembly and reassembly could be accomplished, with a very large effort. In early 1968 it was reported that it is now possible to make many copies of a given piece of DNA; this part of the problem appears to be pretty well licked. It may well be that the most difficult job will be to define what is a "good" gene. At the moment we also do not know how to cut out and isolate a specific gene.

One other problem must be confronted. If we do want to play this game of gene manipulation it is necessary that we recognize that the child will have nothing to say about what it is to be like in life. However, since this is a "minor" problem let's brush it aside for the moment. In fact, we'll come back to a number of other equally "trivial" problems all at once a bit later.

INSPECTION OF THE FETUS DURING PREGNANCY IS A THIRD SERVICE WHICH WE CAN PROVIDE PROSPECTIVE PARENTS. So far, I have described two types of "help"—the prediction of probability that a given set of parents will have a defective child and the chemical correction of defective genes. Both of these methods or services, however, can be effective only for those defects which depend upon a single gene, or at most upon a group of genes that lie close together on a chromosome.

When I received the letter from the mother of the twins mentioned above, I concluded almost immediately that this did not fall in the category of simple gene defects: normally, it takes a gross change in the brain to cause all the defects exhibited by the twins. Accordingly I wrote and asked the mother if there had been complications during the pregnancy.

As I anticipated, she replied that she had hemorrhaged quite severely during the second and third month, just when the embryo's brain and spinal cord are being formed. When I saw this sentence, I jumped to the obvious conclusion that the whole mix-up had arisen because the twins did not have adequate oxygen and/or nutrients just at this critical stage of embryological development. However, two sentences later the mother wrote; "Incidentally, I hemorrhaged quite severely during my second pregnancy. Thus in response to the mother's initial question to me, we didn't know exactly what to advise her daughter, who was about to be married.

It is very likely that the severe hemorrhaging did lead to the abnormalities by causing defects in the development of the brain. By the same token, since the mother hemorrhaged badly during two of her four pregnancies, we must suspect that the hemorrhaging itself may be genetically controlled—in fact, that it may be the result of a dominant gene. Further; a check by telephone to the mother revealed that her own mother, in turn, and also her sister, had been plagued with the same problem. Thus, we cannot tell the young lady what her chances are in any given pregnancy until the second or third month or even later.

Just before Christmas last year I got another long-distance phone call from this family. The daughter, who had been married for almost four years, was now pregnant for the first time and in the middle of the third month had begun to hemorrhage quite severely. Through sobs of fear she told me her story and concern, and then her husband on the extension phone asked, "Are there any tests by which we can determine whether this fetus is or is not going to be normal?"

Unfortunately for their peace of mind my answer had to be, "No, we don't have any tests to give you the information you desire." However, it is entirely possible that this may be feasible within the next ten to twenty years.

In the fall of 1965, *Life* magazine carried a series of four articles on new developments in biology and medicine. In the September

10 issue they showed pictures of how it is now possible in the case of monkeys—not humans—to remove the developing fetus from the mother's womb halfway through the pregnancy, after all the vital organs are formed. Not only is it possible to inspect the monkey fetus at this point, but instruments can be inserted for measurements to be made during the rest of the pregnancy without causing apparent ill effects. Some people argue that we should develop techniques for the use of humans where we suspect trouble such as the young couple have encountered. To a limited extent this is done right now by a Caesarean operation to exchange blood in some human fetuses where Rh problems have arisen.

Actually, it is not necessary to wait for these developments in order to determine some things about a fetus. For example, it is possible right now to test some of its biochemical capabilities.

Near the end of the fourth month, the amniotic sac begins to form. Eventually this "water sac" will occupy a sizable fraction of the volume within the womb. It is a very simple operation to put a hypodermic needle through the wall of the abdomen and remove a small amount of the fluid. Not only can tests be run for the presence or absence of a few critical biochemicals in the fluid itself, but cells which have been sloughed off by the fetus into this fluid can now be grown through a few cell divisions so as to secure enough material on which to perform tests for various deficiencies. As we shall see later, one laboratory has now pinpointed the abnormal chromosomes in a fetus which will definitely produce a mongoloid child, and I have already described tests that seemed to indicate that a child is going to develop amaurotic idiocy.

Ultimately it will be possible to grow amniotic cells obtained in this way into a mass of material approximately the size of the end joint on your little finger. With automatic machines now being developed, it should then be possible to obtain in approximately twenty-four hours an analysis of the ability of this fetus to make any of 200-500 different biochemicals. At the minimum, we hope it will be possible to develop these techniques so that immediately after birth a snip of tissue can be taken from either the buttocks or the sole of the foot, from which we can gain this kind of information for a newly-born child as a means of anticipating the preventive medicine that may be necessary at various stages in its later life.

WHAT DO WE DO ONCE WE HAVE THE INFORMATION? Science is providing us with the techniques for obtaining this crucial knowledge, but science will not tell us what to do. Let us come back, therefore, to some of the "trivial" considerations mentioned before.

Let's suppose that the technique for removing a fetus from the mother's womb is developed, and that ten years from now you are serving along with eleven other people on a jury which meets in a room adjacent to an operating room in a hospital. You are considering what to do about a pregnancy of the daughter of the couple with the microcephalic twins. She is now thirty-five years old, and during the second month of this hypothetical pregnancy she has had severe hemorrhaging. It is now the fifth month, and at the request of her husband and herself the doctor has removed the fetus, measured the head, and—based upon experience of this new technique —is able to say with certainty, "If this child is returned to its mother's womb and allowed to go full term, it will be definitely microcephalic, with a head only about two-thirds the normal size. Like its twin aunts, it will be blind, deaf, and have epileptic seizures. Shall I put the fetus back for the remaining four months of the pregnancy, or shall I abort it now?"

Along with its burdens of conscience, this jury system has a nasty feature. The doctor *must* do one of two things, and so you cannot have a hung jury. You have to decide yes or no. Would you vote to abort this fetus?

Perhaps it isn't surprising that more than two out of three people hearing of this case, vote yes, for this is one of the easiest cases to vote on. Let's go to a much tougher one. On this same day, a lab report comes back on the biochemical capability of cells taken from the amniotic fluid of another pregnant mother. In that case, they suspect the child may have two defective genes for phenylketonuria (PKU).

Children having two genes for this particular recessive trait will not be able to handle properly one of our twenty essential amino acids: phenylalanine. As a consequence, unless treatment is initiated their brain development will be distorted, so that they will have an I.Q. of 20, 25, or at most 30, so that they will never know even who or what they are. Further, these children cannot be taken out in the sun because they are unable to tan properly. And they will have epileptic seizures.

Even if PKU is detected at birth—and most states now require that all newborn babies be tested for it before leaving the hospital —and they are put on a terribly restrictive diet which has essentially no phenylalanine, the best they can hope for, apparently, is an average I.Q. of 100. The exposure to the phenylalanine in the mother's blood stream during the critical stages of brain formation causes irreversible damage. Furthermore, there is strong suggestive evidence that any children of a person with PKU will suffer an I.Q. deficit of as much as 15 I.Q. points.

Another critical consideration is that the diet is really miserable. I was once on it for two days and couldn't wait to get off. The same is true of most of the youngsters: they are always at the neighbors, begging for some kind of food handout. If the neighbors relent and give them even one or two cookies a week, this is probably enough to trigger off brain damage.

Thus we have a trait which is quite serious in its repercussions, not only for this generation but for the next. It is treatable, but the treatment itself is pretty grim, and probably not wholly successful in giving the individual his true mental capacity. Do you vote to abort such a child?

Where this question is put to an audience, usually 10 per cent vote to abort, 25 per cent vote not to abort, and two out of three don't vote. Frankly, I guess I'm one of those "wise cowards" who doesn't vote on this one. Though I feel strongly that a fetus is a life, I would vote to abort the microcephalic child. My Yes vote simply says there are things worse than taking a life so far as I am concerned. However, when we come to PKU, I am no longer clear exactly what it means to be my brother's keeper. If I pay attention only to the commandment "Thou shalt not kill," then I must vote against all abortions. But if I heed the Golden Rule it is quite a different story.

Would you be willing to serve on such a jury? Will your answer change if it requires twelve people, and they can only get eleven others in your community—so that only if you personally volunteer will anything be done?

DO YOU FAVOR GENE MANIPULATION? Suppose I could show you

via a test that you are carrying a defective gene for one of the most common child-killing defects, cystic fibrosis, which is another recessive trait. The child who gets two defective genes for CF will be unable to digest his food properly, but we can now treat this pretty well. In addition, his ligaments won't form as they should, so that he will have trouble using his arms and legs. The lungs will fill up with fluid, and this must be eliminated almost daily with considerable pain to the child. Further, the CF patient is very susceptible to all kinds of infections. Even with the best possible care most of these youngsters will not live beyond their teens. We have a fairly inexpensive, simple test to search for people who have one good and one bad gene for this trait; unfortunately, we get a definite answer somewhere between 40 and 60 per cent of the time.

Let's suppose that you are one of the three out of a hundred people who carry one of these recessive genes. If your partner in marriage is also carrying a matching defective gene, then there is one chance in four that any children you have will end up with this catastrophe. If I now tell you that we have a virus which we feel fairly confident will correct the defective gene, do you want the virus injection?

Do you really know what you voted for? Now that you have voted, I've just *remembered* that I "neglected" to tell you some rather pertinent information about this virus being investigated at Oak Ridge National Laboratory. Quite a bit is known about the arginase molecule, which some humans cannot make (as we saw, apparently the DNA in the rabbit virus carries instructions for manufacturing it). Further, the amount of DNA in the virus is known pretty accurately: there is about five times as much as would be required to specify the construction of arginase. So what becomes of that other 80 per cent of the DNA? In rabbits, it produces an extremely severe and usually lethal skin cancer. We don't know what it may do in humans, although in the somewhat more than 20 people who have been accidentally infected as a result of their research there seemed to be no direct side effects.

This leads to one of those trivial problems. In this case, there was a side effect in the animals, but apparently not in man. The next time it may be the other way around. It is essential to reemphasize that, since the genetic makeup of man is not identical with that of any other animal, the only final test animal for genetic manipulation techniques is man himself. And we can only be secure after 25-40 years when those resulting from a given gene manipulation have themselves had normal offspring.

Suppose, then, that you knew you had a defective gene for cystic fibrosis, and requested the virus treatment which had not caused any ill effects in animals. But now there is a severe side effect in your child. Can you look that child in the eye? Perhaps not. But suppose you knew you had a defective gene and *didn't* try—and then had a child with cystic fibrosis. Could you look that child in the eye every morning for from ten to fifteen years as it wasted away, realizing that you hadn't even tried to save it from its fate?

This is one of those "damned if you do and damned if you don't" situations. In fact, suppose we could develop all these techniques to the ultimate, so that you could now choose everything about your child prior to conception: size, shape, I.Q. potential, color of skin, color of hair, and so on. Would you want to choose your child from a mail order catalog prior to its conception?

If you don't say yes, then let me ask two more questions. Have you worked, or are you planning to work, very hard to give any children you may have the best economic start in life? Have you worked, or are you planning to work, very hard to give any children you may have the best educational start in life? Incidentally, let me point out that the best educational system in the world will be of no benefit to a mongoloid child or one with microcephaly, and if you leave such a child a million-dollar inheritance, it can't legally inherit it. Why not, therefore, work just as hard to give a child the best genetic start in life?

We don't have the power, but suppose we could give you the option of having a child with an I.Q. of 200? This child will not only *think* it is smarter than its parents, teachers, ministers, and so forth; it will be. Would you want such a child?

Would you change your vote if you found that the Russians had solved this problem and were breeding a whole future generation with I.Q.'s of 200?

You laugh perhaps, but you get the point. We can be reasonably sure that initially we will use transforming viruses only to avoid and correct certain kinds of defects. However, once such a technique is perfected at all—considering the pressures that exist in our world —very quickly we'll go to somebody's definition of the ideal man or woman. The problem is Hitler, too, his definition, and I certainly didn't agree with it. In fact, it would be tragic if we were to find only one virus for some very common and pretty uncomfortable defect. Since people would not really have much choice about using it, we might end up with most people looking or acting an awful lot alike.

DO YOU REALLY WANT TO KNOW WHAT YOUR CHANCES ARE FOR PROCREATING A DEFECTIVE CHILD? Suppose that we can develop accurate tests for many more than 19 defective genes. For example, 3 out of every 100 people should have a defective gene for cystic fibrosis; 1 out of 5 should have at least one defective gene for diabetes; 1 out of 70 will have a defective gene for PKU and so on. Would you like to know even before marriage whether you have any one of 100 seriously defective genes?

For the next two or three questions imagine that you are in church—in other words, I want an honest answer! Suppose those tests showed that you and your prospective partner in marriage both have a matching gene for a serious defect—let's stick with cystic fibrosis, since it is fairly common. Your chances of having a seriously defective child if you marry and have children is one out of four. Would you still get married? Under those circumstances would you take careful steps to see that you had no children— assuming that you could adopt? Let me now make one of the most important points of all in this area.

Do you know how many such defective genes each one of us has, *on average?* We estimate that the answer is from 5 to 10. That is, on average each one of us has 5 to 10 genes so defective that if they are matched up by our partner in marriage, then with one chance in four a catastrophe is going to result. Thus we are not merely talking about a poor defective individual in an institution some- where. Each and every one of us is involved in this problem.

Normally the genes don't match up to produce a defective child, because each of us has somewhere between 10,000 and 100,000 genes. But they do match up all too often: 1 per cent of our live births are so defective that they never know they are a human being. That means 40,000 to 50,000 youngsters born in this country every year will never know whether they believe in a God or don't believe in God—they can't form that concept. There is another 1 per cent who are born "nonequal." That is, they are defective enough so as not to be able to get either a job or a marriage partner. For example, a very careful survey was recently made in Boston of 1500 youngsters who were in one or another of the Office of Economic Opportunity programs. Thirty-one per cent had defects so severe that they will be on the poverty rolls from the cradle to the grave—they just can't help themselves. Some had a hole in the septum separating the various parts of the heart; some had vertebrae that had not fused properly, and so forth.

In addition to this 2 per cent there are another 4 to 6 per cent who deviate from what we consider normal. (If you want to know what I consider normal, *it's me*, and I'm not terribly sure about you.) Joking aside, this totals to something between 6 and 8 per cent. In other words, somewhere between one out of every 12 and one out of every seventeen births is defective in some way right now. And the situation is getting worse, not better.

UNFORTUNATELY WE ARE CONSTANTLY INCREASING THE POLLUTION IN THE GENETIC POOL. This pollution is one of the prime examples of how a new finding can be a two-edged sword. Every time we discover a treatment (which is not a cure) for a defective condition, we keep people alive who previously would have died before reaching the age for procreation. Now they live long enough to pass on their defective genes. The discovery of insulin, in other words; insures that the number of people in the population with genes for diabetes will increase. In the past, people who were seriously nearsighted were likely to have an accident before they reached the age to have children; thus the number of genes for serious nearsightedness was kept at a moderately low level. Now we have glasses, and the fraction of children with serious eye defects is on the increase.

I can use myself as an illustration. I am highly allergic to certain kinds of protein. Fortunately for me, they are found only in a very few foods. Some years ago I inadvertently got a heavy dose of this material and went into deep shock. If my wife had not been able to get me to a doctor, I would have died within another ten or fifteen minutes. The doctor recognized the problem and gave me a shot of the right kind of serum to bring me around. But within that same year I passed on one gene for that defect to my son Davey, and four years later our daughter Kim got another.

Probably most of us would agree that once people exist on earth we must try to give them the best possible life. But the real, nagging question is that of the next generation. What obligation do we have to provide them protection?

Some people might argue that we should initiate a program of enforced abortions and sterilizations. While this would give some protection to the next generation, it will not clean up the genetic pool, since each of us still has 5 to 10 seriously defective genes which can be passed on—even though our marriage partner may not have a matching defect, and thus we ourselves do not have a defective child.

Perhaps by this time you are saying, "Well, let's not mess around." Unfortunately, you are over fifty years too late with the suggestion. We have been messing around, and this is why we must now address ourselves to all these problems. It was about 1910 when we turned the corner in medical science to the extent that, if you went into a hospital, your chances of coming out better than when you went in became greater than 50-50. From that time on, we began to tamper seriously with the old law of the survival of the fittest. Accordingly, we face a very unpleasant but crucial set of three choices.

1. We can go on with our present medical practice, but with the clear knowledge that we will have more and more pollution of the genetic pool. In fact, it is now estimated that within five to ten generations (75-150 years) one out of ten children born will be seriously defective in one way or another.

2. We can continue the current medical practice for most people, but make a deliberate choice to reinstitute partially the survival of the fittest by not giving medical care to some defective youngsters, or performing preventive abortions or sterilizations.

3. With all the hazards involved, we can embark upon the road of genetic manipulation.

Unfortunately, there are no other alternatives, so which do you choose? (Normally 5 per cent vote to continue as we are, almost no one wants option 2 and the overwhelming majority choose to proceed with gene manipulation.) It is not enough, though, simply to choose to manipulate human genes. Other complicated decisions must be made also. For example, should gene manipulation be restricted to correcting severe defects, or should we strive to put in some positive attributes? (Positive by whose definition?) In other words, with the background you have so far, would you say that after all these millions of years of evolution man is still not where he should be—that he is not the Godlike creature he might be—and thus we should try to improve him?

WHO SHOULD DECIDE WHETHER A COUPLE SHOULD OR SHOULD NOT GO AHEAD AND HAVE A CHILD? is one of the most critical questions we must face, once genetic information is generally available. Before you try to weigh this question, let me point out that Denmark has already decided that many individuals will not have a choice. They have drawn up a list of defects, and if you happen to have one of them, you can't get a a marriage license until you have been sterilized. (Perhaps I should add that they say nothing about illegitimate children; you just cannot have a legal one.) That is one direction we can go in, with government deciding all.

Do you say no, let's go in the other direction and leave it strictly up to the parents? I suspect your dilemma is similar to mine. Normally, my belief in individual rights would lead me to vote no, but I know of a young lady with an I.Q. of 35—whatever such a low rating means—who married a real budding genius: he had an I.Q. of 50. Recently she had their fourteenth live child. The highest measured I.Q. of the eight oldest children is less than 70, which means that all their children fall in the idiot-or-below classification. Would you say they should not have been allowed to have children?

Also, if two parents beat their child so severely that they cripple it for life, would you say they are not fit parents and the child should be taken away from them? Predictably most people say yes to this question, since we do have laws to this effect and nobody is quarreling with them at the moment. However, suppose that two people with the recessive form of muscular dystrophy marry. In some cases they can have a child, and if so, that child will get two defective genes since both parents have two defective genes. Accordingly, the act of procreation has the same crippling consequences for the child as if its parents had brutally beaten it. Would you say they should not be allowed to have children?

But you will recall that we have a test to determine when a parent has a good and a bad gene for this trait. Suppose a couple do have one chance in four of having a child with muscular dystrophy—should they be allowed to marry and have children?

Yes—where *do* you draw the line? In fact, *who* should draw the line? I trust me to draw the line, but not you, and I suspect you feel the same, the other way around.

A WHOLE NEW PRINCIPLE IS INVOLVED. We believe in our society that once a child is born it has all kinds of rights and privileges. This is what our laws are all about. Moreover, a person like myself, who considers himself slightly conservative politically, is quite shaken to realize that basically our laws say that society rather than parents guarantee these rights. In fact, parents can keep a child, *only* so long as they do not hurt it physically; they can keep a child so long as they give it proper medical care; they can only keep a child so long as they educate it properly; and so on.

We also believe that once a child is conceived it has certain rights. It has the right not to be aborted, except under unusual circumstances. Furthermore in practically every state the fetus has legal rights. For example, if the mother is involved in an accident and the child is born defective as a consequence, after birth the *child* can sue whoever was responsible and can collect. In most states the fetus acquires these rights during the fourth or fifth month of the pregnancy. In my home state of Michigan, we had a recent Supreme Court decision stating that the child has these legal rights from the tenth week of pregnancy on.

An unconceived child, though, is a hypothetical nothing—it is a sperm in a man and an egg in a female—and so has no legal rights. If you ask most any lawyer, he will tell you very quickly that to speak about the rights of such a hypothetical nothing is nonsense. However, we scientists can tell you (according to probabilities) an awful lot about that hypothetical nothing. We can tell you that if it's a sperm in a man with muscular dystrophy and an egg in a female with muscular dystrophy, the child will be crippled, and so on for many kinds of defects. Thus, we must address ourselves to the question that underlies this new principle.

SHOULD THE UNCONCEIVED HAVE RIGHTS? In particular, should some youngsters have the right never to be conceived at all, if they can never possibly know even who or what they are and will only have a life of misery?

Would you say, "Come on now, it is a God-given right to have children, don't play games with that"? If so, then the unconceived child shall have no rights.

Or do you say, "Yes, the unconceived child should have some protection"? If so, then you must take away from parents rights we normally recognize as theirs.

We suddenly have a conflict of rights, and it cannot be resolved with everyone keeping their rights intact. Ten years ago, we couldn't even ask these questions, for we just didn't have the information to deal with them in a meaningful way. Now we do, and now we must wrestle with the nasty dilemmas that come along with the opportunities.

To show you how subtle the problems may be, let me describe briefly a program we have considered initiating in Michigan. Our Genetic Early Monitoring System was devised to aid doctors: you see, 90 per cent of practicing doctors were trained prior to the time that 90 per cent of the information I have given here was available. Further, doctors are terribly busy people often faced with the cruel choice of whether they will treat another patient or read about the newest discovery. To give them help, I recommended that when a doctor diagnoses a child as having any one of the 500 or so defects we know are genetically controlled, he or she should report this on a punch card to a central facility. We would then give back to the doctor the most up-to-date information about additional tests that can be run, both on that child to verify the diagnosis and also on parents or brothers and sisters, to determine whether they are carrying a defective gene. The cumulative information in such a central file could also be extremely useful in helping us to determine whether some defects are or are not genetically controlled.

So far so good. I think probably most people would agree that the procreation of a life, and that they should have the maximum information available as they enter into such a serious undertaking. Now comes the problem. Should we require that the doctor tell each and every parent what is involved or not? For the reasons given, I feel strongly that we should. However, we might pay a rather high price for getting this knowledge out. Parents who are informed will fall into four categories. Some will simply not have enough intelligence to comprehend the information. There will be those who simply don't care, or at least don't want to show restraint. There will be other parents who say, "Okay, so my chances are one in four of having an abnormal child. They are three in four of having a normal one." And they will go ahead. Finally, there will be those who say, "One in four is just too great a chance; I couldn't do this to a child," and they will refrain. Their very restraint is the sort of consideration and commitment which would make them good parents. Thus, the price we pay for such a program is that we remove from the group of those who have children a large number who would be some of our best parents.

In spite of this obvious complication and potentially very high price, I feel we should go ahead with such a program. My reason is simple: I have faith that, properly informed, most people will be responsible. However, if we were to institute such a program, and 25 years from now I found that most people were being irresponsible, then I would change my tune. I simply do not believe that we can disregard the potential rights of that unborn generation. Of course, parents' sense of responsibility may go up dramatically if the principle is established that a child can sue its parents for negligence. A case currently being appealed in the courts may establish that principle.

When I first spoke on this subject, my secretary transcribed some of my remarks from the dictaphone. When she had finished she brought the material in, stood by the side of my desk, slammed it down, and said, "Boy, I'm glad we have had our three children!" I am sure many other people also feel that ignorance is bliss. However, we do now have the information and thus we must ask very carefully, "What must I do to be a keeper of my brothers and sisters yet unborn?"

"Things do not change; we change."

—H. D. THOREAU, *Walden*

✖

CHAPTER 3

Cancel My Reservation, St. Peter, I've Decided To Stay On!*

RED: A person shouldn't be allowed to choose when he's going to die. I believe that when the good man upstairs decides my time is up. He'll simply say, "Come on home, you've done a good job, it's time for a rest."

AUGENSTEIN: I'm a bit perplexed, Red. When you had that bad heart attack last year and your heart went into fibrillation, the good man upstairs was beckoning you home. But the doctor attending you said, "No, no, Lord, not right now," and he opened your chest and reestablished a regular heartbeat. Why didn't you complain then about the doctor rewriting those final travel orders?

In 1963, when I began speaking to groups about the ethical problems arising from scientific advances, I found people often unwilling to believe that many of the possibilities I described would ever be realized. In fact, after those early talks at least a third of the questions from the audiences reflected sheer (or perhaps hopeful)

*This material was first given as a talk at a meeting of the local Council of Churches, Monroe, Michigan, January 1968.

37

disbelief that these new tools would ever come into being—i.e., the momentous new problems would not have to be faced. Over just a five-year period this type of question became markedly less frequent, and then in South Africa Dr. Barnard carried out the first heart transplant. Since then questions of disbelief are no longer forthcoming.

Instead I am asked, "Why can't you keep all the transplant patients alive?"

The heart-transplant operations have pretty well established the idea that science can do presumably just about anything. They have also probably done more than anything else to jolt the public into awareness of ethical and moral problems arising from science. This is one case where limited success has brought really fantastic problems. To illustrate, let me begin by indicating our current capability and limitations in this area.

IT ISN'T THE SURGEONS' FAULT THAT ALL TRANSPLANT RECIPIENTS DON'T LIVE: the progress made by surgical teams in the operations themselves is almost unbelievable. Just twelve years after the first kidney transplant the surgical techniques for kidneys and hearts have become so routine that almost no one dies of the operation itself, though two highly skilled teams must be involved.

The survival problems come about a week later, when the body which has received the transplant suddenly realizes that those new cells don't belong there. As a consequence the body's whole immune apparatus tries to throw out this foreign invasion. If the medical team does not use either radiation or drugs or a combination of the two to greatly diminish the body's ability to make antibodies, the transplant will be quickly rejected. However, if too much of the body's immunological capacity is destroyed, then the patient is unable to fight off infections. Thus, if bacteria invade for which we do not have an effective antibiotic, the individual dies. In fact, this is what has caused most of the deaths following transplants so far. Of course, this is not critical for identical twins, since their cells are exactly the same and thus rejection is not a problem.

JUST WHEN IS A PERSON DEAD? The pinpointing of the moment of death is one of the biggest problems to be faced, because we don't have enough appropriate donors. For example, in the first heart transplant operation carried out in South Africa, this question arose as they considered what to do about treating the young girl who had had a sizable fraction of her brain destroyed in an automobile accident. Although her heart and respiration were still functioning, there was little or no detectable electrical brain activity. It seemed clear to everyone involved that she could not recover, and further, that no matter how long she went on breathing she would never have any mental capability. Further, Mr. Warshkansky badly needed a heart, and it appeared that their cell types were close enough so that there was a reasonable chance of success.

Legally a person is dead in South Africa when the brain has no electrical activity. Even so, those responsible reportedly still asked themselves whether they should use all of the heroic methods available to continue her heartbeat and breathing as long as possible, or do nothing to put off total death. In this case, the doctors and the father of the girl decided just to let the heart and lungs stop naturally.

If you had had to participate in the decision, would you also have voted to turn off the sustaining machines? Suppose no transplant operation were involved—would your vote be different?

In most states in the United States, a person is legally dead when a licensed doctor certifies it. Normally, death is certified when there is no brain activity, no heartbeat, and no breathing; however, a number of doctors have urged publicly that new criteria be adopted. Perhaps a pending homicide case will force a reassessment of our legal definition of what constitutes death.

In 1968 Clarence Nicks was badly beaten in a fight in a bar in Texas. Hours later in Houston's St. Luke's Hospital he showed no electrical activity in his brain and had had no reflexes for hours. Accordingly, the machine which had been providing oxygen to his blood was turned off and his heart was transferred to John Stuchwish, who lived on for quite a few days.

Hesitation was reported as to making the transfer, since the man who beat Nicks was likely to be charged with homicide. Thus there was concern that the *whole* body was legal evidence and should not be fragmented. However, they proceeded with the transplant when the county medical officer agreed not to take action against them for "hiding" evidence.

But this may not be the only legal question involved. Perhaps the trial for homicide may hinge upon whether Nicks was actually dead, since his heart beat on in John Stuchwish's body for an extended period of time. Would you be willing to serve on the jury which decides that case? Those jurors will undoubtedly play an important role in reassessing the legal definition of death.

In this instance, Nicks' brain was so mutilated that it would never function again. Is that a proper criterion of death? Or should a functioning heart also be taken into account?

A suit on a similar issue is now under way in Brazil, where it is reported that a prospective donor who had been the victim of a traffic accident came in with eyes which were completely dilated and faltering breathing, but a heart which was still beating. A tissue test determined that he was a suitable donor, and the hospital had a recipient who very much needed a heart, so the victim was wheeled to an operating room. According to the reports, when the electroencephalograph showed no electrical activity in the brain, the surgeon opened the victim's chest and left it open for over an hour, until the heart stopped. When this heart was put into the recipient, it began to beat immediately without the usual electrical shock. The wife of the accident victim is now trying to sue the doctor for removing the heart without permission.

It is cases such as these that will force some legal definition of just what death is and under what conditions organs can be transplanted from one body to another.

WHO IS TO GET THE PRECIOUS SPARE PART? is another closely allied question. A hypothetical situation will show how tricky such decisions can be.

Dr. Blaiberg, a dentist in his late fifties with a fine grown-up family, was the second heart recipient in South Africa. Although it has been reported that there were a number of people in the hospital who badly needed a heart, Blaiberg was a prime candidate because the rest of the organs in his body seemed to be functioning quite normally, so that the probability that this transplant would work was very great. But suppose one of the other patients had been another professional man who also needed a heart transplant; that he was in his early forties, with young children to bring up; and further, that the cell-matching tests had been equally promising in the two men. Now suppose the latter man had been an extremely heavy smoker, so that he had serious congestion in his lungs and other complications, and the chance of the whole body surviving a heart transplant operation was only half that for Dr. Blaiberg.

Here the choice would be between a man who has lived a full life, but in whom there is a great chance the operation will be successful, and a man whose initial chances are not so good, but who—if he does survive—has more long-term survival potential, both for society and for himself and his family. Do you vote to give the heart to Dr. Blaiberg? Or to the younger patient? Or can't you decide?

A critical question, of course, is *who should decide* who gets this critical organ? Should Dr. Barnard decide? Some might argue that he should not, because he was too emotionally involved to give a rational decision. That is, after the death of Warshkansky, like any normal person he needed more than anything else a success, so that he probably would be heavily weighted toward a patient like Blaiberg. Before we disqualify too quickly Barnard or his counterpart in any given situation, though, we must remember that it is he who will wield the knife, and thus it is he who must bear the consequences of any failures.

Kidney transplant operations have brought on some unexpectedly tricky dilemmas. I have already described the tough situation of the twenty-two-year-old grandson and his sixty-six-year-old surgeon grandfather. Since the operation was performed successfully, there is now a chance that the grandson's other kidney may go bad while his grandad is still alive (as we noted, the probability for this may be much larger than normal, since the grandfather's kidney breakdown appears to be a genetic defect). If so, does the grandson have either a legal or a moral right to get his kidney back?

Recently I was told of two men who drew up a trial contract dealing with a comparable situation. The one, who has had complete kidney failure, offered to pay $10,000 to the other man for one of his. However, the contract was not for an outright sale, but rather for a lease arrangement: accordingly, it specified the physiological conditions which would be defined as nonfunction of the remaining kidney in the donor, and thus give him the right to retrieve his leased organ. According to the report I received, a circuit court judge gave an informal opinion that a person could sell or lease any real property which he owned, but not irreplaceable parts of himself. Other opinions are reportedly being sought on this question, and I don't know what the final outcome will be.

There are also numerous reports of perfectly legal situations where the transplant recipient and/or relatives suffer severe repercussions. I talked recently with a couple where the husband had received a kidney from an accident victim. Once it was decided that he should receive the next transplant, the couple had to move into an apartment right across the street from the hospital so as to be immediately ready for an operation when a kidney became available. Unfortunately for them, none was at hand right away, with the result that every time the couple heard a siren they began to hope subconsciously that this would be an accident victim who would die right in the hospital under ideal conditions. As a consequence, two very fine people began to view themselves as ghouls: they knew what was happening, and why, but were unable to stop it. Now, I doubt whether they will ever be able to pick up the pieces and totally rebuild their shattered self-respect.

Some recipients of kidneys are reported to suffer severe depression and guilt feelings. The same is true for some people on kidney machines. The reaction in both cases appears to result when they get help while others die because of an inadequate supply of spare parts or facilities. Accordingly, the question, "What made me so much more worthy than the others?" begins to nag at them.

Clearly, we all hope that we can minimize some of these dilemmas by finding ways of greatly increasing our supply of spare parts. We may be able, eventually, either to trick the recipient's body into not rejecting organs even from animals, or to make synthetic parts, or perhaps to take cells from a person's own body and make new organs—either one at a time or in groups. Let us look briefly at the problems in the first two methods before considering the last possibilities in greater detail.

THE ORGANS OF A NUMBER OF ANIMALS HAVE SIMILARITIES TO THOSE IN MAN. For example, one man survived for a few months on two chimpanzee kidneys. The Russians have been arguing all along that we should not use human hearts for transplantation, but rather calves' hearts, since they are the proper size. We already have a glimmer of hope that we may in the future be able to change the surfaces of cells so that the host body will not reject a transplant organ. The problem can be stated fairly straightforwardly.

The molecules on the surface of any cell appear to be arranged in a fairly specific mosaic. That is, the different classes of molecules are arranged like a giant jigsaw puzzle. Although the picture for a given cell appears to be fairly definite, in theory the basic building blocks or pieces can be put together in an almost endless number of combinations. Thus, in many cases cells from two different bodies may be so different that a tremendous immune response arises. However, mosaics on the exterior of cells from near relatives should have a number of common features, since many of the genes that control the surface are from a common source. Of course, with identical twins the surfaces are the same, since the genes controlling them are identical. If we could now find some means for changing the mosaics on the exterior of heart cells coming from a calf, then presumably the human body would not recognize these as being different, and therefore would not reject the transplant.

It is possible by various treatments to change the exterior of the single-celled animal, Paramecium. Apparently the chromosomes in these cells have the capability of specifying quite a spectrum of mosaics (at least 10), so that, depending upon the environment, different exteriors are selected. Whether something similar is possible in mammalian cells, so that cell surfaces can be changed chemically, is simply not known.

Another technique offers a different promise. When portions of the surface of cells are digested off by enzymes, cells from different individuals will fuse for a time, during which the chromosomes from the two cells apparently intermingle. Although eventually there is presumably a resegregation of the chromosomes, the new cells formed may not have the same complement of chromosomes as before, so that the cell surfaces of these cells now may be different from the original mosaics. Whether this can be controlled sufficiently so that we can fool the immune response in a human into not rejecting a calf heart is not known. Certainly, there appear to be great chromosome changes in the cells of tumors and cancers, but the host body does not reject them. Thus, many of us are watching further exploration of these techniques with great interest, since this could provide a tremendous increase in the number of organs available for transplanting into humans.

MECHANICAL DEVICES SUCH AS THE SUPPLEMENTARY PUMPS DEVELOPED BY DEBAKEY PROVIDE ONE WAY TO GET AROUND THE SHORT SUPPLY OF HEARTS. However, it is not clear for how many other organs we can build substitutes. Although the heart seems to be the easiest to supplement or bypass, it is not inconceivable that substitute stomachs and perhaps even intestines could be constructed: recently a metal ball and socket was put in place of a hip joint destroyed by arthritis. Unfortunately both lungs and kidneys, because of the need for tremendously large surface areas across which diffusion can occur, pose large technological challenges. Further, we probably will not be able to make a substitute brain in the foreseeable future (although judging by their performance on one of my recent exams, some of my students might be well advised to volunteer for the first tests).

The advent of the bypass pump for hearts, however, posed a troublesome problem in even DeBakey's first operation. Unbeknownst to the surgical team, a blood clot broke loose in the patient just prior to the operation. Moreover, the kidneys and lungs were both seriously defective because of the longstanding medical problems of this patient. The rest of the body simply quit living, but the bypass pump beat on. And as DeBakey said in a nationally syndicated story, he determined when this individual was legally dead by giving instructions to turn off the power to the pump.

In a sense, we are back at the same problem mentioned above when we were speaking about donors. Just what is death? More particularly, just what is life?

IF EVENTUALLY WE CAN TAKE CELLS OUT OF A PERSON'S BODY AND IN A TEST TUBE GROW A NEW ORGAN, we shall have developed one of the most promising methods of minimizing the shortage of organs. Further, when the replacement organ is put back, the body will not try to reject it because the cells belong there. To do this we shall need to overcome some quite formidable obstacles, but again, we can at least see what has to be done. The situation is as follows.

At conception, when the sperm and egg united to form that fertilized egg from which each of us arose, all the information needed to specify every detail about us was there in that single cell. However, as it divided to give 2 and then 4 and 8 and 16, 32, and so on, some of the information was disregarded as the cells began to differentiate. There are now some very crude estimates that to become a heart cell requires that the cell pay attention to only about 20 per cent of its total information, and to become a lung cell, it pays attention to a different 20 per cent, and so forth. The remaining 80 per cent appears to be put away in storage somehow. The fact is, we have some inkling as to how this information is "turned off." The trick would be if we could grow cells in a test tube and get them to go back and pay attention to the information they once had. For it is now possible to grow some human tissues in tissue culture through approximately 10 cell divisions during which the chromosome number remains at the normal 46; but then in later divisions the number may jump to 80 or 120. To reconstitute an organ will require that the cells grow normally through approximately 30 cell divisions, and it is important to emphasize that the last 20 divisions will be a lot more than twice as hard to control than the first 10. Even so, we have material to work with.

Recently a number of laboratories have been able to chemically alter the differentiation pattern in both plant and animal cells. To change a given cell's pattern of growth requires changing the spectrum of its protein synthesis. This can be done in many cells by the addition of hormones. In fact, even a "salt shock" can be used to change the spectrum of ribonucleic acid templates (needed in protein synthesis) produced by individual chromosomes.

Suppose that we can learn how to make new organs by controlling differentiation. (I think I am pretty safe in betting that we shall be able to remake at least hearts and livers within this century.) Let's look far ahead at the implications. Suppose that three hundred years from now you go in for your 320th or 330th or 340th annual checkup, depending upon your age, and the doctor says, "You're in good shape, except your third liver is going bad. Let me take a snip of tissue and come back in a month when I've run it through thirty cell divisions, and I'll plug in a new liver." But you think for a minute, and say, "Well, no—I don't think I want it this time. I thought it was a pretty good idea the first two times we played the game, but a hundred years ago I had a bad psychological experience which my psychiatrist hasn't been able to get me to forget. I've lived a full life. No thanks. This time I'll call it quits."

If, in fact, we can perfect this technique, your refusal would be tantamount to committing suicide. In other words, to choosing your time of dying. If we can provide an almost indefinite life-span, should people not only have the right to choose to live, but also their time to die? Would you say an individual should have the right to choose his time of death?

If your answer is no, then let me ask: Just what is immortality? Is it to consist of an indefinite stay here? Or is it something reserved for a good place in the life hereafter? This issue cannot be disregarded if we can begin to give people an almost indefinite stay of life.

Perhaps if you said people should not have the right to choose to die, you felt that this would be contrary to the biblical statement that "the Lord giveth and the Lord taketh away." Yet by the same token, if we prevent death by an organ transplant, we certainly are not letting the Lord take that life away according to his schedule. I had a typical conversation with a man on one of my television shows, of which an excerpt stands at the head of this chapter. When I asked him whether he felt a person should have a right to choose his time of dying, he said no. This was surprising to me, for I knew he had had a serious heart attack and had been brought back to life at the last moment, when the attending doctor opened his chest, stopped the fibrillation of his heart, and started it beating again electrically.

I'll never forget the look on Red's face as he suddenly comprehended for the first time what had really been involved in the doctor's action. With an air of complete amazement he said, "You know, I never thought of it that way." And so it is with people in many walks of life, now that we have at least partial control over life and death.

SOME OF THESE AND OTHER TECHNOLOGICAL BOTTLENECKS COULD ALSO BE REMOVED BY MAKING CARBON COPIES OF OURSELVES. This possibility comes about from recent research on frogs. In this work an "incision" was made in a frog's egg and the experimenters removed the nucleus (which contains only the mother's one-half of the normal number of chromosomes). This was discarded and replaced by a nucleus (containing the normal number of chromosomes) taken from a cell elsewhere in this frog's body or some close relative. Placing this mature nucleus into the remaining immature cytoplasm of the egg resets the clock—so to speak—and the whole assemblage behaves like a newly fertilized egg. Accordingly about 5 per cent of the time a perfectly normal frog is produced. The actual probability of success depends upon the cell from which the new nucleus is taken—if it is taken from embryonic tissue, then the nuclear transplantation is almost 100 per cent effective.

To do this in humans would require that we surgically remove an egg from some woman's ovaries and discard its nucleus. We would then take the nucleus from a cell (probably one of the crypt cells in the intestine) in the person's body we want to duplicate and put it in the cytoplasm of that egg cell. This "newly fertilized egg" would then be placed into the womb of some woman wanting a child who had received appropriate hormones so that it implants properly in the wall of her uterus and nine months later we have a carbon copy of the person from whom the critical nucleus was taken. It is important to emphasize that the term *carbon copy* is precisely correct because the new individual now has chromosomes identical to the original donor—they are indeed identical twins in all respects except age.

At the moment attempts at nuclear transplantation in mammals are quite unsuccessful. However, if all the problems can be solved, this option would be a God-send for couples who have seriously defective genes. For example, any children procreated by the two couples mentioned previously who each had a good and bad gene for either amaurotic idiocy or muscular dystrophy will be afflicted with one chance out of four, whereas a carbon copy of either parent would of course be normal.

But suppose a person contracts for a carbon copy and then at birth puts it in the deep freeze as a source of spare parts. Now if he (or she) needs a new heart they simply thaw out that particular frozen organ and grow it through three cell divisions (instead of thirty) so that it is the proper size to fit their adult body.

Assuming we can solve all of the technical problems, do you think this is a good idea? Somehow not many people are enthused about this particular option. And properly so, because now we are dealing with a new individual.

But really what is an individual? Does a brain define the individual? Certainly if you were to put Einstein's brain into an athletic, adolescent body tremendous changes would undoubtedly occur so that you would no longer have *the* Albert Einstein. This question of what constitutes an individual, of course, underlies the dilemmas posed throughout this book, and in particular those in this chapter.

What makes one individual worth more than others so that they should get a critical spare part or be the one to get onto a kidney machine? When has a life been fulfilled so that that individual should be allowed to go meet St. Peter?

DOCTORS AND NURSES CONTINUALLY FACE THESE KINDS OF CHOICES. I listened recently to a neurosurgeon describing to a group of nurses the intricacies of a particular type of brain operation. To make his point easier to follow, he described the operation as he had performed it on a particular patient. After giving all the pertinent details from his notes, he then went on to list some of the extra procedures he had taken to minimize any brain damage. As it became obvious that he was coming to the end of his presentation, he said, "As you people know, I am not one to brag, but I think technically that was the finest operation I ever performed: in fact, it is probably technically one of the best, if not the best operation I have ever participated in or witnessed. Unfortunately, I wish I hadn't been so successful, because the patient is now paralyzed from the neck down. I certainly didn't do that boy any service by saving his life."

His remarks struck an extremely responsive chord in me, for when I was in the Army Medics I was instrumental in saving the life of a boy who also became a vegetable. I was the corpsman who rode ambulance one evening to an accident where a soldier had been thrown from a jeep and hit his head on a rock. I used all the procedures prescribed in the manuals to keep him from bleeding to death before we reached the hospital and then scrubbed in and helped on the operation. Unfortunately, he reverted to the behavior of a four-month-old child. What a sight to see them change the diapers on this 6-foot, 180-pound body—!

It is painful to remember the look on the faces of that boy's parents when another corpsman and I brought him home. The outer shell of their son was changed only slightly, but the insides were scrambled beyond recall.

I had been instrumental in saving a life. But for what?

Nurses in intensive care units are perhaps most often hit by decisions of this type. If one of their heart patients goes into fibrillation, or if another patient will die if he doesn't get a respirator, the nurse has less time to decide what to do than it has taken to tell the above story. Deterioration begins in a brain deprived of oxygen for more than two or three minutes, and a person in whom circulation stops for from six to eight minutes will be a vegetable if he or she can be revived at all.

What should the nurse do if her initial treatment isn't immediately successful? For example, would you want to be revived if your heart had been stopped for four minutes, so that you would almost certainly suffer fairly serious mental defects?

Perhaps most importantly, are there situations where emergency treatment should not be initiated at all? Suppose a microcephalic child only a few hours old was in your care and needed a respirator to survive. If you turn it on you know this child will survive, but be blind, deaf, and have epileptic seizures. Would you turn the switch to ON?

Suppose you were responsible for a five-year-old microcephalic child who only weighed 17 lbs. because it screamed for most of the twenty-four hours. Would you deliberately not start the respirator?

Well, this situation actually arose. The nurse wouldn't "be responsible for making a decision that would cause someone to die." Thus, when she did turn the switch, the one chance for that child to die legally passed, and as a consequence the poor kid has screamed on now for five more years with no immediate end in sight.

Would you start the respirator for a child with amaurotic idiocy?

Would you turn it on for a ten-year-old child with cystic fibrosis who has already begun to degenerate?

Would you turn it on for an infant with PKU who must live for years with that miserable diet just to retain that fraction of his native IQ capacity which has not already been destroyed?

Again let me emphasize that the nurse has far less time to decide than you have taken to answer. But although doctors and nurses are on the firing line every day, few of us can really escape these decisions. I am sure you recognize that we should be facing these questions openly right now because of the many advances in science which are keeping people alive longer and longer. In many cases the medical techniques really don't prolong life, but just postpone death.

MOST FAMILIES HAVE HAD A LOVED ONE IN A TERMINAL ILLNESS AT SOME TIME, AND THUS HAVE HAD TO ASK: WHAT IS THE MOST HUMANE THING TO DO—keep my mother or father alive through continuous suffering, or let them slip on their way mercifully and with dignity? In my own family we have had to face this question with three of my four grandparents. Most recently, my grandmother at the age of eighty-nine went into a coma rather unexpectedly. The doctor called my father, who was her only living child, and stated that perhaps by using heroic methods he could keep her alive a few weeks or months, whereas if he made her comfortable she would live at most a few days. Since she had deteriorated badly both physically and mentally in the last few years, and was obviously unhappy in life, my father told the doctor to make her comfortable. When Dad called and talked to me about it, I immediately concurred, for Grandmother had been extremely unhappy for quite a few years.

Would you have agreed under the circumstances with our decision? In fact, do you think that such a decision should be made by immediate members of the family? Incidentally, there was a fairly large estate involved here. Yes, that does make a difference, doesn't it? However, I can assure you that the money was never a consideration. But this is not always true.

In many cases when such a decision has to be made, economic factors cannot be disregarded. Probably most people know of some example or other of a mother or father who has had a very serious illness, which was obviously going to be terminal in the not-too-distant future, and where if they used all possible methods the family would be put irretrievably in debt. In fact, I know of two cases—one involving the mother and the other the father—where if everything possible were done to keep them alive for an extra six or nine months, the children in the family probably could never afford to complete their education. In another case, a family went desperately in debt to keep the grandmother in her seventies alive for an extra six months. To pay off the costs both the mother and the father of three little children held two jobs for a period of about six years, just when those youngsters needed their parents at home. Eight years later, two of those children are in correction homes.

Who should make the decision in instances such as these?

Laws and practices are quite confused in this regard. I know of instance after instance where either the patient or the patient plus the immediate family have pleaded in vain with the doctor or the hospital to let the patient go on his way. One of the worst examples involved one of my colleagues. A few years ago he invited me to his home one evening, along with two other friends, and related the following story:

"My father is in a hospital in another state and is obviously in a terminal case of cancer" (from his description of the symptoms, it was obvious there would be no miracle recovery in this case). "They give him sedatives every four hours, with the result that he is comfortable for one hour, wakes up and is fairly lucid but very uncomfortable for a second hour during which he pleads to be let go on his way, and then essentially goes out of his mind for the remaining two hours. We have asked the doctor not to treat him any longer and just to let him go on his way in a relatively short time. However, the doctor insists on proceeding with his treatment and predicts that Dad will live for at least another three months. He told us quite candidly he wouldn't stop or delay treatment, since if his colleagues were to review the way he handled this case and felt it was improper he could lose his hospital privileges. In fact, he told us another doctor had lost his hospital rights for precisely this reason in a neighboring county just a year or so before."

I asked my colleague why they didn't take the father out of the hospital. He felt this was impractical since the father's hospital was over five hundred miles from the home of his nearest son or daughter and there were no other adequate facilities to care for him nearby.

"Further, to keep Dad alive requires fairly frequent transfusions. When these were first begun we had to sign a release, and so we have now told the doctor we want to revoke that permission. However, he told us that the hospital would probably get a court order to continue. The problem is that a few years ago they heeded the demands of a mother—because of her religious belief—not to give her child a needed blood transfusion. It died. The father, who was separated from the mother and did not share her religious convictions, sued the hospital and collected a large sum of money. Thus the hospital itself will take no chances. But the doctor has told us quite pointedly that next weekend all the judges will be out of the county, because of the long holiday, and so no court orders could be issued. What ought we to do?"

Would you have advised them to halt the transfusions? Well, they agreed with the way most people vote, and Dad did go on his way. Recently when I was in that town I checked the obituaries in the newspaper. About three times as many older people died on that weekend as on the following two weekends combined. Perhaps it was chance, but I doubt it!

Whether you agree or disagree with what was done, I trust you agree that this is an awful way to do business. If people are not to be allowed to choose their time of dying, then plug all the loopholes. If they can choose, then let them do it in a straightforward, open, but above all, carefully controlled fashion to avoid six million being sent on their way by a future Hitler.

THE CONSIDERATIONS I FEEL ARE MOST CRUCIAL IN THIS GENERAL AREA WERE PERHAPS BEST SUMMARIZED BY A PRIEST FRIEND OF MINE. This man was responsible for hospital practices in one of the largest metropolitan areas in the country a few years ago. After much soul-searching and a fair amount of bitter controversy with some of his colleagues, it was decided that when a person comes into one of the hospitals in his jurisdiction who either is rational and makes the proper request, or (if he is irrational or in a coma) for whom the family makes the proper request—and if it is deemed a terminal case by three staff members in that hospital—then they will not make a pincushion out of this patient. Instead, they give him the last rites of the church, make him comfortable, and wish him a good journey.

As I sat talking with my friend late one evening, he said that the controversy over whether they should or should not use this procedure had been so bitter that it was obvious they would never get unanimity of agreement. And since he was responsible for the hospital practices, the decision basically became his to make. He explained the reason for it as follows: "I decided that I was willing to go meet my Maker with it on my conscience that I had allowed ten or perhaps even a hundred people to die the day before a miracle cancer cure was discovered. But I could not go to meet my Maker having it on my conscience that I had kept thousands or tens of thousands or maybe even more people alive through endless suffering, waiting fruitlessly for the cure that never came."

This pretty well sums up the thinking that must go on, not only on the part of individuals but by our society as a whole, now that we have our newfound capabilities. What does it mean to be my brother's keeper, now that I can control to a remarkable extent my brother's coming and going?

If the world were not so full of people, and most of them did not have to work so hard, there would be more time for them to get out and lie on the grass and there would be more grass for them to lie on.

—D. R. MARQUIS, *The Almost Perfect State*

✖

CHAPTER 4

Our Exploding Challenge*

To put one's finger on the one problem facing mankind which overrides all others is simple. Unless we solve the population explosion, we can forget about the rest.

THE MAGNITUDE OF THE POPULATION EXPLOSION CAN BE ILLUSTRATED BY A VERY FEW FIGURES. The average increase in population per year throughout the world is 2 per cent. (Most of us have either mortgages on our home or savings accounts, and so we know there is a formula for computing compound interest which tells us how much money we either owe or will have at a given time. The same formula can be used to compute exactly how many people there will be at any given time.) If we continue to increase at 2 per cent per year, the world population will double in a short 35 years. In other words, we will go from more than 3 billion people now to almost 7 billion by the year 2000. If we continue to increase at the

*The material in this chapter was first presented in a university course and as a public lecture at Msgr. Gabriels High School, Lansing, Michigan in 1964. It is available on a 16-mm film from the Audiovisual Department of Michigan State University, East Lansing.

same rate for 500 to 600 years, there will be one square yard per person over the whole face of the earth.

Perhaps we should look further at this staggering number. For example, all of the more than 3 billion people alive on the earth today could be packed—one per square yard—within the confines of metropolitan Chicago, and almost 1.5 billion could be put into Detroit and its suburbs. But bear in mind that at our present rate of growth this would be the situation, not in a few Chicagos and Detroits, but over the whole face of the earth, including deserts, mountains, polar icecaps, and oceans. And this not in some dim, incalculable millennium, but in a few hundred years—hardly longer than from Columbus' first glimpse of America to the present day.

If we still did nothing about slowing down the increase, then in another 1700 years, at our present rate, the sheer physical mass of people would exceed the mass of the earth itself. And if we continued to give people platforms in space from which to procreate, in about 6,000 years the mass of people would exceed that of the known universe.

Such figures become absurd, and it is hard to believe that we will not find adequate solutions to the problem fairly soon. But let us not underestimate its seriousness. The solutions *are not yet found* so far as active application is concerned, and even in thirty years the situation can become desperate as to food and other aspects of human functioning, to say nothing of international pressures. Unfortunately, there is nothing hypothetical about these numbers; either we stop the annual increase or these will be the levels of population.

One other point must be emphasized here to lay the basis for discussion. The 2 per cent per year figure is an average value—it is not uniform throughout the world. In the "Western" world—which includes Australia, New Zealand, western Europe, Canada, and the United States—the increase is just about 1 per cent a year; in Russia, southern and eastern Europe, Japan, and Argentina, it is about 2 per cent a year; while in the rest of the world, which encompasses two-thirds of the world's population (i.e., in the rest of Asia, all Africa, and the rest of Latin America) the increase is almost 3 per cent a year. At a rate of 3 per cent increase per year, the previous numbers become 23 years for doubling, approximately 350 years for achieving a density of one person per square yard, about 1200 years for population to exceed the mass of the earth, and about 4000 years to exceed the mass of the known universe.

Costa Rica, for example, has one of the most serious rates of increase—about 4 per cent a year. At this rate, their population will double in less than 20 years. The doubling time for Mexico at the present rate of growth is about 23 to 24 years: in fact, if they maintain their existing rate, there will be one billion people in Mexico in approximately 125 years.

THE CONSEQUENCES OF THIS TRAGIC EXPLOSION ARE MANY AND VARIED. Perhaps just three different considerations will serve to illustrate the size of the problems generated by it.

Food. There have been numerous reports in the newspapers and on TV that two-thirds of the world's population goes to bed hungry every night. In fact, half of the world's population is in a serious condition of malnutrition. Some experts in agriculture claim that if we really made an all-out effort for 25 years, we could increase our food productivity sufficiently so that the number of people now in the world could be fed at the minimum level we consider adequate for nutrition. This would mean a crash program to raise the productivity of lands now being tilled and also to bring perhaps as much as 50 per cent of new land into production. (Many people don't realize that normally it takes fifteen to twenty-five years just to get new laboratory findings out into the fields.) The bitter truth is that even if we make such an all-out effort—almost like the Manhattan Project to perfect the atomic bomb—but do not have a moratorium on increase in population, the number of people will just about double in that length of time, and we shall either be worse off than we are now or at best keep even.

Two specific examples further illustrate this point. We all know what a fantastic achievement it has been for the Egyptians to build the Aswan Dam. The waters backed up behind that structure can be used to irrigate new lands and thus increase food production by an estimated 20 per cent. Unfortunately, the increase in population in Egypt during the building of the dam will be essentially 30 per cent. Thus, in spite of one of the most momentous engineering feats of all time, when the dam is finished the Egyptians will actually be further behind in feeding their population than before they started. I have noted above the fantastic increase in population in Mexico. They are already irrigating a larger fraction of their arable land than we are in the highly developed United States. Unfortunately, they cannot increase production further in this way without extensive desalinization of water, since they do not have additional water resources to tap for irrigation.

Industrialization. Most of us would be delighted if some way could be found to industrialize the have-not nations. Let's see how feasible this is for just one country. India now has approximately 600 million people. Almost 400 million of these are in agriculture. To have a truly industrialized nation, not more than 25 per cent of the people can be "down on the farm"; in the United States, for example, only about 5 per cent of the population is now involved in agricultural production. Thus, to industrialize India just to the minimum extent would require the creation of at least 250 million jobs. To create a job in this country costs on the average about $50,000. Taking an optimistic view, it may perhaps be possible to create new jobs in India at an average cost of about $3,000 per job. Thus, the total cost for India would probably be at least $750 billion. This represents the total gross national product of our own country for one year. Unfortunately, since India's GNP is only about $20 billion per year, $750 billion represents about 40 years of India's total GNP. It is important to point out that Hitler and Stalin with all their repressive measures were never able to reinvest more than about 25 per cent of their GNP. At that rate, it would take India almost 150 years to invest the required amount in industrialization.

Clearly, this is an almost hopeless task. And even if, by some miracle, they could reinvest their total gross national product for 40 years, they would just be able to industrialize *for their present population*. During that time their population would have more than doubled, and they would then need more than 500 million new jobs.

Overcrowding. Urgent as food, industrialization, waste disposal (pollution), and water supply, etc., may be, many of us think that the most critical commodity will be simply living room. Even though we can never allow this to happen, let's see what the figure we are actually heading toward—one person per square yard—

would mean in living conditions. (I must emphasize once again that *no effective brake* has yet been found to reduce the actual rate of increase, so that this figure is what we are heading for.)

One way of stacking people in, one per square yard, would be to build apartment houses 100 feet on a side, put five families to the floor (each family of four would have about 1,000 square feet, or a smallish 6-room apartment) and make the buildings 50 stories high. On this basis, we could leave 100 feet on all sides for recreation, communication, transportation, and a vacation perhaps once every hundred years or so (if everyone tried to go to the seashore at once, we would have a uniform layer of almost a thousand people deep all along the United States ocean front). Perhaps if we programed our playgrounds very carefully, boys between the ages of eleven and sixteen might be allowed to play basketball for an hour a week.

The obvious question arises: What happens when you crowd people into such a limited space? For good reason, experiments have not been run with human beings under these conditions in a controlled way, but the results from some well-controlled animal experiments cause many of us to be deeply concerned. Perhaps the most instructive experiments were run with white rats at the National Institutes of Health.

The experimenters built four very large pens with runways connecting the various enclosures. In each of the enclosures were comfortable nesting areas and sleeping quarters for the animals. To begin the experiment, equal numbers of males and females were placed in the experimental area. Very quickly, the two biggest meanest, toughest males "set up shop" in the two end pens and established nice, well-run harems—they could do this because they could sleep at the foot of the runway coming into the two end areas, and when an animal tried to come down the runway females were allowed to pass, but males were chased back. Within a short time, however, massive problems became evident in the two center pens where there was a predominance of males. In fact, the experimenters compiled a long list of neuroses.

The easiest of these to catalog was the abnormal sexual behavior. For example, when the females came into heat, the males would pursue them relentlessly until finally the females literally dropped from exhaustion. During the subsequent pregnancy, these animals would not establish nests, but at delivery would drop their pups at various places in the enclosure and walk off and leave them—the mothers couldn't care less. Although food was never in short supply, the other animals would cannibalize the newborn.

Experimenters also observed homosexual behavior between the males, and the males would try to have intercourse with the females in the center pens even when they were not in full heat. None of these things happen in a well-run colony.

It's a long way from an animal population to a human one—or is it? If you take the list of neuroses which experimenters observed in the center pens and go to our big city ghettos, you can check them off one at a time. Thus the nagging question is, "Just how far is it from a rat population to a human one?" In other words, can you really crowd human beings indiscriminately without encountering the same kinds of problems? For example, if we stacked people in with the same density as prevails in Harlem, all the 200,000,000 people in the United States could be put into the metropolitan area of New York City. Guess what would happen then!

THE CAUSES OF THE POPULATION EXPLOSION ARE SURPRISINGLY SIMPLE. In this connection science has really been a two-edged sword: we have tried to utilize its fruits in a humane way and in so doing have generated this most inhumane situation. Put succinctly, we have become too fruitful and multiplied too fast. Again let me illustrate.

As nearly as we can tell, throughout most of recorded history there have been about 40 births per thousand of population per year and just about as many deaths. In fact, in the time of Christ the average annual increase in population is estimated to have been about one-tenth of one per cent, at which rate the world population took a few centuries to double. But during the industrial revolution, beginning in the 1700's, we began to clothe, feed and house people better, and as a result the death rate began slowly to decline, until by 1850 it had dropped to 30 deaths per thousand per year. When you subtract this from the estimated 40 births, you get an average increase in population of one per cent per year. This was approximately the rate up to 1914, and during those 60 years the world population essentially doubled.

Then at the end of World War II, we invented antibiotics and began to apply them throughout the world, with the result that the average number of deaths has come crashing down to 12-16 per thousand per year (in the United States and western Europe this ratio is already down to 6-9 per thousand per year). But at the same time, world-wide births have only decreased to an average of 36 per 1000 per year. Subtracting the number of deaths from the number of births gives the current number of 2 per cent per year as the average world increase in population. The alarming thing is that the end is nowhere in sight, for not only has the total population exploded, but the average rate of increase has gone up so that even the catastrophic figures given at the beginning of this chapter may be overly *optimistic* unless population control programs are initiated almost immediately. Moreover, breakthroughs which will appreciably increase the availability of human spare parts may lead to an additional lowering of the death rate in medically advanced countries, so as to further aggravate the worldwide increase in population.

Thus, the population pressure will undoubtedly force us to reassess how long a person should live. Clearly we cannot allow our population to go on increasing very much longer: ultimately it must be held constant at some number. The only real way to do this is to allow a child to be born when somebody dies. Cruel as this may sound, it is really the only way to make absolutely sure of holding things level. Furthermore as will be emphasized in the next chapter we must control population within the next 25 to 50 years, and organ transplants will probably be perfected for at least some of our organs within that time.

Perhaps the way to put the problem most starkly is as follows. Suppose we have come to the situation where we must hold the population level by permitting conception of a child only when someone dies. Thus, if a grandfather or grandmother gets a heart, liver, or kidney transplant, then their grandchildren cannot get a permit to have a child. If an argument were to develop between the two generations involved, who should win? Do those already here have squatter's rights? Or do the children still to come have rights.

Would you say that the grandparent should win? Or should the grandchildren?

Unfortunately, most people who hear this question posed sit and laugh and refuse to vote either way. Yet the situation may be not more than twenty-five or fifty years down the line, so we had better do some pretty fast thinking on it.

The storage of people in the frozen state on a mass scale could compound the pressures even further. I have no enthusiasm whatsoever for this development, but a number of groups have already begun to freeze people either just prior to death or immediately after. When the bodies are maintained at the very, very low temperature of liquid nitrogen, all cellular processes stop and the person is truly in a suspended state. These groups recognize that during the freezing process there will be a lot of little icicles formed which will punch holes in cell membranes causing a lot of cell damage. They argue, however, that because of the rapid rate of biological progress, in a hundred years or less we will be able to thaw the frozen people and not only undo the damage caused by the freezing process, but in fact correct whatever caused their death. For example, they claim that with cancer they will be able to completely cure the cancer and put people back into the pink of health just as they would have been in youth.

I repeat that I do not share their enthusiasm, for with the population explosion we certainly don't need another source of people. In fact, so far, there can be essentially no controversy over the points I have mentioned since there is nothing theoretical about the figures —the straightforward calculation simply shows what numbers of people will result if we continue at our present rate of increase. Certainly no thoughtful person can look at these numbers or even briefly consider the consequences without saying this cannot be allowed to happen. It is essential that we all look carefully at possible solutions. I shall examine these in Chapter 5. In fact, an important point can be made by disposing of one suggestion immediately.

EXPORTING OUR SURPLUS PEOPLE HAS BEEN ADVOCATED IN THE PAST BY A NUMBER OF PERSONS WHO SHOULD HAVE CHECKED MORE CAREFULLY BEFORE THEY SPOKE. They have argued that we ought to follow the example of Europe during the great days of colonization—that is, export people to "new worlds." Although such a proposal may sound attractive, even the following simple calculation would have shown, not only that such a scheme cannot work, but that the proposal should not even be expressed, since it may mislead some people into believing we can avoid facing up to the tough decisions that must be made.

From consideration of the available food, water, and living room, and the problems of waste removal, it is often concluded that we dare not let the world's population go beyond 10 billion people. At our present rate of growth we will reach that number in about 50 years. If at that time we still had a 2 per cent increase each year, it would then be necessary to export 200 million people annually. Needless to say, this is a very lage number (the size of the present population of the United States), and so even if neighboring planets were habitable, we would quickly overrun them and have to look for room in other solar systems. We suspect that there may be many planets very similar to earth, since some nearby suns wobble in their paths apparently because of the attraction of satellite planets which we cannot detect with our telescopes; and a planet has actually been observed revolving around one of the closer suns.

Thus, to make our calculation let us assume that the nearest star to us, Alpha Centauri, does have a planet similar to earth. This star is 4.3 light years away. (Remember that light travels 183,000 miles per *second*. A light year is the distance it travels in a *year*.) The fastest any of our interplanetary probes has traveled is 10,000 miles an hour. Let's assume that with new technological advances we can achieve speeds of 1,000,000 miles per hour (this increase by a factor of 100 would take some first-class development during these 50 years). At that rate, it would take about 3000 years to enter the solar system of Alpha Centauri.

If people refuse to practice strict birth control here on earth, it is unlikely that they will do so in a space ship. If we started (very hypothetically) with two people and maintained an average increase in population of 2 per cent per year for the 3000 years, the space ship would contain 100,000,000,000,000,000,000,000,000,000 people at the end of the journey. This means that we would have to launch 100,000,000 space ships a year (that is, 3 per second), each holding two people at the start but ultimately capable of containing a total population equivalent to 10,000,000,000,000 present earths. It is an interesting thought.

The obvious absurdity of these alternatives should sober us. As devices for pampering ourselves to simply not facing the awesome problem before us, they are little short of criminal indulgence in unreal fantasy. The problem is not only at our gates; it is already costing the suffering and death of some *millions* of human beings every year, with incalculable repercussions on international politics from the rising pressures involved in a great many areas. Clearly, if we do not surmount this fearful dilemma, it will almost surely be the explosion that so poisons our Garden of Eden that no one can be fruitful in any endeavor any more.

And God blessed them, and God said to them, "Be fruitful and multiply, and fill the earth and subdue it; and have dominion over the fish of the sea and over the birds of the air and over *every living thing* that moves upon the earth.

—Genesis 1:28

✖

CHAPTER 5

The Monkey on Our Backs*

The facts already presented leave no doubt that the population bomb must be defused immediately. Nevertheless, some still try vainly to hide their heads in the sand. Unfortunately, there are those who misuse the scriptures by citing only that small fraction of the verse above which says, "Be fruitful and multiply and fill the earth," in the hope that this gives them license to refuse to face up to reality and their responsibility as intelligent human beings. As one man said, "I don't think we should do anything! The good Lord put me here, and the good Lord will look after me."

Certainly, I believe that the good Lord put me here, but he also gave me a mind so that I would pay attention to all parts of Genesis 1:28. Each of us must realize that in the past animal populations

*The material in this chapter was first presented in a University course and as a public lecture at Msgr. Gabriels High School, Lansing, Michigan in 1964. It is available on a 16-mm film from the Audiovisual Department of Michigan State University, East Lansing.

have been controlled in *only* three ways: by (*a*) starvation—and as I have already indicated, we hope that with a moratorium on population increase we can lick this problem—certainly no humane person could choose to solve the problem of population increase by allowing malnutrition to become even more rampant than it is now; (*b*) pestilence—the use of antibiotics which has wiped out plagues of all types has really spawned the population explosion; and (*c*) by predation—man is his own predator in terms of war.

Most who have studied the situation carefully are very fearful that unless we do something on a world-wide basis before we have 10 billion people, the pressures will become too great and once again man will prey on man in terms of a nuclear holocaust. The tragedy is that even such a stupidly catastrophic solution to the problem would be only temporary: even if the war were to wipe out 50 per cent of the world's population, we would come right back to our previous population level within 35 years if we still had a 2 per cent annual increase in population. Thus, if we refuse to use our brains to avert this kind of catastrophe, some idiot must push the button every 35 years or so.

For the above reasons, we must insist that *all* men use their individual minds in time to institute a fourth method of control—some form of *rational* control. After all, we are one of the living things that moves upon the earth, and thus we must have dominion over ourselves.

Whatever we choose to do, the method must bring births and deaths into balance if population is to be held constant. We must either increase the death rate or decrease the birth rate: these are the only two alternatives.

INCREASING THE DEATH RATE IS NOT VERY ALLURING TO MOST OF US.* Yet a few countries have been using what one may consider an increase in death rate to control their population—they have legalized abortion. For example, Japan has held population growth under 2 per cent a year by government licensing of a million abor-

*One of my students suggests that the way to solve the population problem in the United States is to give everybody down to the age of twelve a driver's license *and* a car. Another suggestion is that if all smokers would inhale while they smoke five packs a day, the increased death rate would just about bring things into balance.

tions a year (they recognize that probably more than two million occur).

Although some countries favor the use of abortion to solve the population problem, I do not. According to my ethical code and that of many others, it is simply a form of increasing the death rate, and thus not appropriate for solving *this particular problem*—particularly not on a world-wide basis.

THE BIRTH RATE CAN BE DECREASED BY A NUMBER OF METHODS. For the moment let us consider only their efficiency and explore the moral implications later. *Time* magazine in the summer of 1964 had an excellent brief summary of the effectiveness of various approaches to the problem. They pointed out that if 10,000 normally fertile women, living with their husbands and undergoing normal intercourse, practiced no birth control, 900 of them would become pregnant during a year. This is the normal fertility rate.

The *rhythm method*, though it may have some moral virtues, is not very efficient. That is, even if the same number of couples refrain from intercourse for from three to five days in the middle of the menstrual cycle, 400 will become pregnant. The problem is that ovulation in the ovaries is not wholly regular. There is in fact a suspicion now that intercourse may actually trigger off ovulation in some cases.

This method also has another serious flaw in terms of world-wide effectiveness. In the underdeveloped countries where population control is most needed, many women cannot count accurately. Some population control groups have tried to circumvent this problem by distributing strings of twenty-eight beads to the native women, with five beads of one color for days when there was to be no intercourse, and twenty-three of a different color for the remaining days in the menstrual cycle. This attempt, however, was often thwarted because many of the women rearranged the beads into more artistic designs.

Contraceptives are efficient enough to solve the problem. If either the husband or wife uses mechanical contraceptives or foams according to prescription, about 100 will become pregnant within a year.

The *"pills,"* when used as directed, are quite efficient. 100 out of

10,000 would become pregnant in any given year. In fact, it is found that almost always the 10 who do conceive failed to take their pills for one reason or other for too long a period and then tried unsuccessfully to double up later.

There has been considerable controversy about the possible side effects of birth-control pills. For example, there have been reports that women taking the pills had blood clots. These seem to be true, but often the reports fail to mention that women the same age who are not taking the pills also have blood clots—apparently with about the same frequency. Further, it is not absolutely clear just how long women can take them; since they are an extremely potent female hormone. Most doctors prescribe that women take certain of the pills for only four years maximum, although other versions are recommended for ten years.

A very few women also become more prone to hysterics; however, this can usually be corrected by changing to some slightly modified form of the hormone. This does suggest a practical precaution, though. A girl who is planning to get married and use the pills should start a few months before the ceremony. In this way, if it becomes necessary to change to a different form of the hormone, it can be done before the couple starts their maximum period of intercourse.

It is important to emphasize that, although there may be a few complications from the pills, they appear to be far less than the hazards of the pregnancy which may result if they are not used. Specifically, 3.2 mothers die for each 10,000 live births in the United States, and other complications which are not fatal occur at a rate probably ten times as high. Further, this risk is greatest in our inner-city areas and in the underdeveloped parts of the world.

The *interuterine insert* (IUI) is one of the oldest methods, rediscovered. It was recorded on ancient Egyptian papyrus that various materials inserted into a woman's uterus prevented conception. This was rediscovered by experiments on animals in the late 1800's.

Specifically, if a small spiral of plastic or metal is placed in the uterus of the female—of any animal—she will not conceive during the time it is in place. Once the spiral is removed, however, apparently her normal fertility returns. Thus the method is reversible. Moreover, it is efficient, since most women can retain these spirals almost indefinitely, although a few will go through a false labor at the next menstrual cycle and expel them. Of this latter group, many will retain the spiral if it is reinserted once or twice.

For world-wide use this method has a number of advantages in terms of efficiency and ease of use. Of great importance—where necessary—the device can be inserted by a person with approximately the training of a midwife, and if a small string is attached, the woman using it can inspect herself periodically to insure that it is still in place. And, as mentioned above, it is reversible: that is, if a woman has two children, has an IUI put in place, and then loses her children through accident or disease, the spiral can be removed and her normal fertility will return.

Sterilization is another method which has been used to some extent in a number of countries, particularly India. This method is, of course, efficient, but has two serious disadvantages. First, it is irreversible in a large fraction of the cases. Second, to sterilize the men will not necessarily solve the problem. For example, if 90 per cent of the men were sterilized, but there was not perfect fidelity between the men and women, the other 10 per cent could carry on their own population explosion. A woman, however, should only be sterilized by highly skilled people under very sterile conditions. Even if we chose to attack the population problem by this route, we do not have a sufficient number of trained persons or facilities adequate to do the job on a world-wide basis.

One other method needs to be mentioned in jest. A number of years ago a woman from the Planned Parenthood League was speaking to a women's club. At the end of her speech, a lady in the audience said, "You make it sound so difficult. Aren't there any simple ways of preventing conception?" After some thought, the lecturer said, "Yes, there is. Drink a glass of water." The questioner looked perplexed for a moment and then asked, "Before or after?" Back came the answer: "Instead of." I don't recommend this one for efficiency!

As you can now see, science brought on the population explosion by giving us tools for maintaining good health, and science has provided us with the methods for halting it. However, as is immediately apparent, science cannot tell us by which specific approach we should attack the problem. Clearly, a number of obstacles must be surmounted before it can be properly resolved.

UNDOUBTEDLY ONE OF THREE ALTERNATIVE SITUATIONS WILL ARISE:(1) We won't use our fifty years of grace to advantage, and with 10 billion people the pressures will become so intense that somebody will push the button, and we will have a nuclear war that no one wants; or (2) we won't use the 50 years to get a world-wide consensus of opinion on how to limit population, but will realize that we are generating a war and will have abrupt, dictatorial control (in other words, every woman will be allowed to have only two children); or (3) we will be able to get the world public properly informed and solve this problem on the basis of individual restraint. Clearly, the latter alternative is the ideal all of us would prefer— I am sure no one wants a policeman in every bedroom. The obvious big question, though, is: How can the necessary information be disseminated in time throughout the world?

In this connection, many people are unaware that the population explosion is producing illiterates faster than the literacy programs are producing people who can read. The fraction of literate people in the world is actually declining, in spite of some rather heroic efforts on the part of educators. Accordingly, we can't publish a two-page document in Washington and expect to solve the problem with that alone.

THE NECESSARY INFORMATION CAN BE DISSEMINATED IN TWO WAYS. One is to educate all the people in the world so far as possible. This is an extremely formidable job: of the more than 3 billion people, approximately 1.8 billion are either in the Communist bloc, where they probably wouldn't welcome our educational programs, or in the Western world, where presumably the educational level is adequate. But this leaves 1.2 billion people or more to be educated. The average life expectancy in the underdeveloped parts of the world is about 40 years. Thus, if we provided ten years of education to all people, we would have to educate a quarter of them, or 300 million people, simultaneously. If we tried to maintain the usual 30-to-1 student-teacher ratio we would have immediately to find 10 million new teachers.

Such a large number of teachers cannot be had by a snap of the fingers; thus we must have some form of mass education. Unfortunately, we don't know whether this is possible without securing the answers to three very big questions. The first is, "Can we train people with teaching machines or area-wide television who have no tradition of the values of education?" If, in fact, this is possible with some village elder sitting in the corner and saying, "Keep busy," it is still not feasible to program all the required material in the almost infinite number of dialects in the world. Thus the second question: "Can we teach these people to read a cosmopolitan language such as French, Spanish, or English within six months to a year?" And even if this were possible, it still is not practicable to design a separate educational program for Nigeria, one for Pakistan, still another for Okinawa, etc.; we must be able to design a core curriculum for the world, with only a few modifications for local needs.

If all three of these things can be accomplished, we can make crude estimates of how much such a mass education program should cost. Actually, various kinds of estimates all give about the same result of $10 to $15 billion per year. The simplest estimate to make is as follows: in this country, it costs an average of about $500 per year to educate a student. In the underdeveloped world, the average cost of living is about a factor of 10 less than it is here, so that it should cost about $50 per student per year, or $15 billion per year for 300 million students. To put this into perspective: this is about the amount the United States spends for health, education; and welfare; the interest on our national debt is also about the same; it is a little more than twice what we spend each year for our agricultural programs (about 50 per cent of which are designed to stimulate production and the other 50 per cent to get rid of the excess); and it is about one fifth of our defense budget. Although this is a very large sum, we must ask ourselves very seriously how much more will we have to spend for defense in the future if we do not provide this kind of education throughout the world.

Certainly ten or even five years of education for all the people in the world will not guarantee us peace and the solution of all our problems. However, I think most of us are convinced that *without* education, we shall be in even more serious trouble than we are now.

A SECOND WAY TO DISSEMINATE THE NEEDED INFORMATION IS ON A SHORT-TERM, CRASH BASIS. Instead of trying to provide general education to all the people in the world, suppose we provide information only on the population crisis and what to do about it. India early recognized the problems brought on by high illiteracy. Initially they tried to get around it with posters. On one side was a picture of a family with two children, neatly dressed, obviously well fed, alert, and very attractive. On the other side of the poster was a family with ten children, dirty, disheveled, potbellied from malnutrition—very unattractive. The reaction of the Indian people was unexpected. Many said quite simply, "Oh, those poor people with *only* two children!" Their tradition, in other words, is the same as our own—Grandma brags about how many grandchildren she has!

The most successful efforts at informing the people of India have involved agents serving dually as agricultural experts and population-control helpers. The agricultural agents went into the villages to help the people increase their food production and gain their confidence. Then, when they saw a woman walking along with a child clinging to her dress, another in her arms, and often she herself pregnant, they would ask, "Do you want to have more children?" Invariably the woman would answer, "No." But it turned out that most women did not know that children are produced by intercourse. With the dissemination of such rudimentary information, plus knowledge of how to avoid conception, one individual was able to get quite significant results in lowering the birth rate in a given village within three to five years. The problem is that there are over 500,000 villages in India alone, and probably at least 3 million in the whole world. Just think how much effort has gone into our Peace Corps, involving only about 100,000 people, and the fantastic energies involved in mobilizing 13,000,000 men and women during the World War II. Even if it only cost $1,000 a year to put a population agent in the field, the total cost would be $3 billion. But again, how much must we spend in the future if we don't invest this large effort now.

AN UNBELIEVABLY TIGHT TIMETABLE MUST BE MET, even assuming we can disseminate the needed information. As I have indicated, we must have a world-wide solution within 50 years, before we reach the overwhelming number of 10 billion. In fact, those who argue about the matter disagree only as to whether we dare not go beyond 5 billion, 10 billion, or 25 billion. The first we will reach in about 20 years, the second in 50 years, and the third in a little over 100 years at our present rate of growth.

If 50 years is correct, then we must look critically at how decisions have been made in the past. In general, when a big issue comes before Western society, it takes about 25 years for the public to become acquainted with the problem and another 25 to set up the machinery and crank out the decisions. Civil rights is a good example: Marian Anderson was invited to the White House in the middle thirties, the Supreme Court decision came in the middle fifties (a little ahead of schedule, according to this timetable), and if we can get out of the civil rights mess in an honorable, humane way by the middle eighties most of us will be very pleased. In fact, the whole question of population explosion seems to be following the same pattern. However, we must bear in mind that this is the timetable for a culture in high levels of education and almost instant communication. Can the same schedule possibly be met for the rest of the world—particularly in its underdeveloped areas?

THE BIG PROBLEM IS TO RESOLVE THE ETHICAL AND MORAL DILEMMAS. So far I have pointed out that there is a growing awareness of the population explosion; further, more and more people are becoming aware of the consequences inherent in this problem and are determined to attack it, using the methods science has provided us for controlling the number of people. However, even if we can perform the technical feat of getting the information out in time, we still must face the most critical aspect: the ethical and moral problems involved.

Unfortunately, I am afraid that most of the present discussions of morality are misdirected, because they deal primarily with which methods we shall or shall not use. For example, I am a practicing Protestant. Accordingly, since as far as I am concerned abortion is taking a life, I believe this is not the best way to solve this particular problem. However, I am perfectly happy with the idea of interuterine inserts, pills, contraceptives, and the rhythm method *providing they are used in a wholesome, responsible way among married people.* But some of my older Catholic friends come along and say no to a number of these methods, because of their moral beliefs. Much as I respect their right, in fact their obligation, to act on the basis of their beliefs, I repeat that these arguments seem to me not directed at the main issue.

Let me use my own set of beliefs to illustrate the point. As I have indicated, I am against abortion but in favor of the IUI. We now suspect—although we are *not* sure—that with the spiral in place the sperm and egg do unite, so that fertilization takes place, but the egg does not implant properly in the wall of the uterus; perhaps this is because of abrasion or pressure exerted by the insert. Let us assume, for the moment, that this is true, and you can see my difficulty very clearly. For me to be in favor of the IUI I must say that at the time of conception the living cell is not sacred and therefore can be prevented from developing, whereas to rule out abortion I must say that three to five months later that life is now sacred, and we should not do away with it simply to hold down population. This is indeed a dubious distinction to make.

However, we must all recognize that the end result of every method mentioned—including the rhythm method—is that some human life does not come into being. And this is where the discussion must be directed. "Which child shall not be conceived so that other children already here can have a fruitful life?"

At least two or three criteria could be used for such a selection. For example, every woman could have two children and then use some means—morally acceptable to her—to see that she has no more. This scheme has the virtue of democracy. A second alternative would be to get even better methods of predicting when defective children will be born and then encourage women to use some method, acceptable to them, to see that they are not conceived. This is very attractive to many people who say that we must reduce our increase in population on a world-wide basis by 2 per cent; this is just about the number of children who are born defective. However, as we have also seen, this means that someone must decide what is the ideal man. A third possibility would be to sterilize everybody, create "perfect" babies in test tubes, and then give each couple two children. Being a natural-processes man myself, I don't view this with great enthusiasm. But these examples are not chosen at random. Each has virtues, each has drawbacks.

It is not my purpose here to argue for or against any of these criteria. My main point is that we must discuss and decide which ones we want to follow. Otherwise we will proceed on a hit-and-miss basis, which is dangerous when the stakes are so terribly high.

LET ME SUMMARIZE THE SIX CRITICAL ACTIONS WE MUST TAKE TO CONQUER OUR EXPLODING CHALLENGE.

1. We must pledge to face up to the horribly tight timetable already djscussed. Let me further illustrate this by a personal incident. In 1964, my wife and I attended an international conference on the population explosion. During the second day of that conference, a Protestant really raised Cain with the Catholics for obstructing progress.

A priest then arose to defend the actions of his religion as follows. "All too often you Protestants are extremely arrogant. Thirty years ago we couldn't have held a conference on this topic. You Protestants appear to have moved more rapidly than we Catholics from this extremely rigid position. You appear to be fifteen years ahead of us. Give us time to examine our consciences."

At this point a genteel lady from India could restrain herself no longer and arose and said, "Sir, if you ask us for fifteen years you cannot have it. In my country, fifteen years from now, at our present rate of growth we will have 200 million new mouths to feed."

As my students say, "There is the whole ball of wax in one story." Here is one of the most critical decisions our society will ever have to face. We dare not walk over the moral scruples of an important minority in our country. By the same token, we dare not let a minority veto absolutely needed action. How do we resolve this problem? More particularly, how do we resolve it *in time?*

2. In the next 25 to 50 years we must undoubtedly negotiate treaties between countries as to the levels of population that will be allowed. Perhaps you may say this is going too far. Yet before you become adamant in that opinion, consider what will happen if all the countries in the world practice population control except the Red Chinese. Yes, we will have to have treaties!

The big questions will be: On what basis do we assign the levels of population? Is it to be so many people per square yard? Or will allowable populations be based on food production levels? Will some insist on striking a balance between the races?

And how shall we police the agreements? What will we do with countries that cheat? Obviously, such treaties must be policed every bit as carefully as the nuclear test-ban treaty yet I honestly don't know what we are to do if a country does cheat. Do we go in and kill off certain number of their people to make them fulfill their obligations?

3. We must provide foreign aid to countries which request it for controlling their population. India and Pakistan asked this country in 1956, not only for information about contraceptives, but also for the contraceptives themselves. As far as they were concerned, these were a morally acceptable method and would do the job in time. Eisenhower, a Protestant, refused this help because he said it would be repugnant to our Catholic citizens. This seems ironic, for while Kennedy—a Catholic—was in the White House, United States counterpart funds were used to foster birth control.

We are all aware that there are many moral codes in the world. And we must not dictate to any country how they will go about controlling their population. Thus, I believe we must insist that they choose some method which is morally acceptable to them, and then provide the necessary help. Certainly it does little good to help a country update its industrial capacity or provide its people with food, unless we also help them control their population. For example, India is trying desperately to increase her gross national product by 5 per cent a year. Yet the population increase is almost 3 per cent a year. Would you advocate that since we do not have limitless funds, the United States should provide foreign aid only to those countries which have effective population control programs under way?

To some my next statement may appear cruel, but I feel it is fundamentally humane. I think we do no service to any country if we go in with antibiotics to save lives and don't at the same time help them control their population. During a recent discussion, Congressman Garry Brown (R-Mich.) and I agreed that the United States ought to insist that countries receiving gift food from us should be required to set aside at least 20 per cent of the equivalent value in counterpart funds to train and support their own nationals as joint agriculture and population-control experts. Unless we attack this problem in at least these two ways, our present good intentions in giving medical aid may actually aggravate and prolong the existing food crisis.

We must also realize that the United States is the only country with the facilities for providing help throughout the world. India, for example, is trying to get a million IUI's in place in their women each year for the next 10 years, so as to bring their population into balance.'However, to manufacture, distribute, insert, and inspect each spiral requires about $6: in other words, $6 million per year. To us this is a trivial sum, but for a country with about three times as many people and a gross national product which is only one-thirty-fifth of ours, it is a large outlay. Unfortunately, the United Nations is not an appropriate agency to carry out such a program. Such action would be taken through UNESCO, and that organization has as many vetoes as there are member states. In fact, the head of the subcommittee on population problems asserted a few years ago that "there is no problem."

4. Since the United States is the only country with resources to attack this global problem successfully, we must select our national leaders with care. They must be men who will address themselves responsibly to the challenge and seek compassionate moral solutions of the problem in time. Above all, we cannot tolerate the irresponsibility of the public official who asked a Brazilian audience what was the matter with them that they didn't have as large families as he did. What made the episode almost incredibly tactless is that northern Brazil has struggled bitterly against tremendous odds to conquer an extremely explosive population situation.

5. The fifth thing we must do is to realize that we may soon have a big problem here at home. Although the present rate of growth in the Western world is only 1 per cent annually, this is probably misleading. Most of the women now having children were born in the late thirties—the depression or the early war years when our birth rates were extremely low. With the post–World War II crop of babies now forming their own families, I am told that within the next 10 years the number of child-bearing females will increase by 30 per cent. Unless they show more restraint than has my generation, we will be off to the races in the Western world also. Although

many hospitals have been converting their maternity wards to other uses, most are making very sure that they can switch back easily and quickly if the pills don't hold the birth rate in check.

6. The final action needed is by far the most crucial. We must switch from a negative to a positive approach. Throughout I have been careful to proceed as we all do today, namely, in the negative vein. In other words: Which child shall not be conceived? Which method shall not be used? As we know from history, invariably the negative approach generates more heat than light. If we continue so, it will be tragic. Rather, we must switch to the more positive question, "Under what conditions should a human life be started at all?"

From the foregoing it should be crystal clear that we *must* begin to limit the number of people on our earth. God has said, "Be fruitful and multiply," but he also said, "Have dominion over all things of the earth"—and I am sure this means that man is meant to discipline himself. Thus, if we must begin to restrict population, and if we have the ability to predict which children will or will not be defective—then *all* parents must ask themselves very carefully, "What should this child be like that we are going to bring into the world? Faced as we are with these possibilities, it is a pity that all too often the procreation of a life is one of the most haphazard of events, and one in which we determine little about its outcome beforehand. Few people, I am sure, would think of investing $50,-000 in a business on the basis of five minutes' discussion. Yet—disregarding for the moment humanitarian considerations—someone must invest between $30,000 and $50,000 in a child if it is to have any hope of success, and many, many children are conceived with far less than five minutes' serious thought. Is this how we should go about the most sacred of all human interactions?

It appears fairly certain that within the next 25 to 50 years we shall have the tools available to control conception much more deliberately and easily. For example, at least one laboratory thinks it now has a preparation which will give a woman permanent contraception as long as she desires and can be reversed easily upon request.

This new possibility works on a principle different from the others. Prior to ovulation the cervix, which is the purse-string muscle at the juncture of the uterus and vagina, secretes a very thin fluid which allows sperm to swim freely into the uterus—some believe it may even attract them. Later in the menstrual cycle the cervix changes, and a viscous material is secreted which is essentially impervious to sperm. Not only has a hormone been found which causes the viscous material to be secreted continuously, but there are chemical variants of this hormone which go into solution very slowly, over a period of years. With proper development, we may now anticipate that a woman who desires it can have a pellet of this material inserted under her skin by a simple operation. So long as it is there she will not conceive. If she changes her mind, the residue of the pellet can be removed—again by an almost trifling operation—and the hormone will be flushed out of her blood stream in about a month, so that her normal fertility should return.

The fears that have attended the increasing use of other devices of less easy and sweeping effect are intensified by this idea. Some people claim that potentially it could destroy our society by permitting anyone to be completely promiscuous without having to pay a penalty. In fact, some say it will destroy our moral code by removing the fear of pregnancy. If so, then I say, "Let's destroy that code, for it is not worth preserving if it is only based on the fear of pregnancy." Some, I am sure, would certainly use such a preparation as a license to drag the finest and most tender of all human acts, intercourse, completely into the gutter. However, I am convinced that such pessimism is selling our younger generation short—I have great faith and confidence in their basic integrity and virtue. Considering that when most of us grew up it was difficult to be immoral, whereas today it is often difficult to be good, I am continually amazed at how many really fine, truly moral college students I encounter each year. While those who are promiscuous appear to indulge more frequently and openly, I really don't feel that the fraction of such students is much higher than in years past. Considering today's temptations, the large number of kids who take morality—in its broadest sense—seriously is an impressive record indeed.

Thus, I am sure that most young couples will welcome the opportunity to spend the first few years of their married lives achieving not only economic stability but also the emotional harmony between husband and wife which a child must find if it is to thrive after it is born. To many it will become abundantly clear that intercourse does and must serve more than one purpose, and that one of its major functions is to promote love and stability in the home—as, indeed, even the beautiful lines of the age-old marriage service suggest.

The population explosion is our largest and most worrisome and demanding human problem. If we handle it badly, then there is no sense in worrying about the others. We must use this problem as the spur that forces us to face up to the question, "Under what conditions should a human life be conceived?" If—and only *if*—we take this positive approach will mankind get a bonus: we shall begin to seek out our divine purpose in a meaningful way.

Were half the power that fills the world with terror,
Were half the wealth, bestowed on camps and courts,
Given to redeem the human mind from error,
There were no need of arsenals or forts.

—HENRY WADSWORTH LONGFELLOW,
"The Arsenal at Springfield," 1845

CHAPTER 6

*The Last Sanctuary**

In chapter 1 we saw that it is now possible to manipulate at least a few of an individual's basic concepts, and thus potentially to control still another aspect of the quality of his life. Just how far those preliminary experiments can be extended is not known, for most experimental psychologists and practicing psychiatrists are very reluctant to really take a person apart and put him back together as would be required in research on mind manipulation. In fact, some people hold that we should never tamper with a person's beliefs, for what goes on inside his head is really his own business and only his. Rather, they say, we should concern ourselves exclusively with his behavior, since this alone is what ultimately affects society. Thus they urge that we should only try to change "abnormal behavior."

There is now considerable evidence that people's behavior can be

*This topic was first discussed with a group of college counselors meeting at the University of Michigan in 1964.

programed fairly easily. The basic premise underlying much current research and development work is that man is after all an animal, and many features of his learning and behavior are very similar to those found in a large number of animals. Hence, they argue, it should be possible to train a human by the same methods that have been so well developed for animals such as rats, dogs, and pigeons.

DRASTIC CONDITIONING OF HUMAN BEINGS SEEMS TO HAVE ITS GREATEST VALIDITY IN THE CASE OF SERIOUSLY ABNORMAL PEOPLE. For example, autistic children show very little normal human behavior: these youngsters are completely withdrawn, do not talk nor respond in any predictable way. And sometimes they are so self-destructive that they don't just chew their fingernails they literally chew their fingers off, and if they are left to run free they will bump into things on purpose or gouge their faces with their fingernails or other sharp objects. Even when they are restrained by a strait jacket, they will bite pieces out of their shoulders if they are free to turn their heads.

These youngsters are totally unreachable by normal methods of love and compassion or even punishment. Many are the firstborn in a family where the parents simply do not know how to treat them. They are apt to reward or punish the child unpredictably for doing essentially the same thing at different times. As a consequence the child becomes totally confused and does not really know what is right and wrong behavior. Dr. Ivar Lovaas at the University of California at Los Angeles has been working with a number of these and other abnormal children, using electrical shocks as a means of conditioning. He put these youngsters barefoot into a room with a metal grid in the floor. Periodically, he gave them a shock which they could avoid only by throwing themselves into the arms of an adult. After a few shocks they quickly began, not only to seek out adults, but to treat them in a reasonably affectionate way.

The experimenters also kept some of the youngsters very hungry and then rewarded them with ice cream whenever they threw their arms around the neck of another child. Quite soon they began to interact meaningfully with other children.

An adaptation of these same techniques, using an electric cattle prod instead of the electrified floor, was employed with a young boy who had been strapped to a bed for seven of his eleven years. As soon as he was turned loose he tried to take a bite out of his shoulder. Before he could close his teeth, however, he was given a severe electrical jolt with the cattle prod. He looked around in a most startled fashion, paused for a few seconds, and turned again to take a bite. The second jolt made him look warily around the room and pause for approximately a minute, at which point he hesitantly began to take another bite. The third jolt was enough— he never tried for another bite of himself while he was under the care of this doctor. Using shocks from either the cattle prod or the grid in the floor, it was possible to get this boy to interact with adults and with other children so that they could begin to train him in a more normal way.

After this very promising beginning, he was returned to his old ward in the hospital, and within a matter of a few hours he was back to his previous behavior. When the doctor visited him there he spotted the problem immediately. As soon as the child tried to take a bite out of himself, the nurses would immediately run up and grab him, and hug him. What they were doing was to reward and perpetuate his abnormal behavior.

Normally, we would classify electric shocks by a grid to the feet or by cattle prods to the behind as cruel. Yet in this case love misapplied had created tremendous problems which apparently could only be corrected by fairly painful measures or not at all.

Clearly, either this type of behavior manipulation or the manipulation of people's basic concepts can produce tremendous good or tremendous damage. Thus it seems critical to ask two kinds of questions. First: What do we know about the mind? So that we can begin perhaps to understand how and why these manipulation techniques work and how they can be developed and perfected. Second: What do we want to do with this knowledge and these capabilities?

To "brainwash" a person requires that we get the desired information in, persuade him to store it away so that it is called upon in preference to other information that may be there, and finally motivate the person to act on the basis of this new information or training. At the moment, our knowledge of all three phases is much more fragmentary than we would like. However, it seems worth-while to mention at least a few studies in these areas, to indicate both what we do know and pehaps more importantly what we don't know, so as to provide some indication of the probable direction of future research.

THE INTAKE AND PROCESSING OF INFORMATION BY HUMANS IS SIMILAR IN MANY RESPECTS TO THAT OF COMPUTERS. In my own laboratory we have found that people performing simple, well-learned tasks, such as playing the piano, typing, adding up numbers, proofreading, and so on have a definite capacity for processing information. In all these tasks, the maximum rate at which our human subjects processed information corresponds to the making of 20 to 30 yes-no decisions per second. In only one study, of highly trained people recognizing words artificially put in random order, were rates approaching 50 yes-no decisions per second reported. Even so, compared to a computer which can make close to a million binary decisions per second, this is fairly slow work. On the other hand, we humans are much more versatile than the most sophisticated computer available or planned.

Further, studies have shown that this capacity is not restricted by our ability either to take in data or to respond once a decision is made. In fact, studies involving the flash recognition of complicated displays exposed for only very short moments of time have shown that a person can take in more information during a flash of only 1/25 second than he can process in a whole second. Studies in other laboratories indicate that the eye can do this from 4 to 5 or more times per second even during normal reading. Apparently the eye takes quite detailed snapshots a number of times a second of what is going on around us, so that we have far more information than our processing unit can utilize most of the time. The information from these "snapshots" is presumably stored away in an extremely short-term memory for a quarter of a second while the data are processed.

In all our studies we utilize random music or random texts, etc., so that our subjects could not depend upon something they might remember from the past, but rather had to process new impressions of each and every symbol. However, if we allowed them to memorize even our random material, it was possible for them to increase their performance in many cases by a factor of 2 or 3. Thus their rate of response—the act of playing a note or pressing a typewriter key—also was not the limiting factor in the process.

The thing that seems to impose the major limitation on our ability to process information is our internal computation unit. In studies involving a variety of tasks we found that humans do not make decisions continuously, but rather in a periodic way like a computer. However, instead of taking only a millionth of a second, one of our computational cycles takes a hundredth of a second or longer. But this is a bit misleading, since from what we know about brain structure, organization, and function, activity involving many, many nerve cells is probably required to arrive at a safe and secure yes-no decision.

The next question is, where and how is this information stored away?

HUMANS HAVE AT LEAST TWO OTHER MAJOR FORMS OF MEMORY which are of concern to us here. Once information is processed, it appears to remain in a short-term, easy-access memory bank for anywhere from 5 seconds to 40 minutes before it is then stored away in a long-term memory, where it resides for periods of the order of 100 years. As I get older, though, I am not quite so sure of this latter number. Thus, it seems worthwhile to indicate some of the experiments that have led to these general conclusions.

For many years a number of psychiatrists have treated certain kinds of psychiatric disorders with electroconvulsive shock. In this case an electrode is placed on each temple of a patient and a powerful surge of current passed through the brain. It is so potent that the patient is knocked out and recovers only after an extended period of time. If the clinician asks him the next day whether the electrodes were cold or were pressed too tight, or if the cot was comfortable on which he was lying, invaribly the answer is, "What electrodes?" "What cot?" In fact, the patient has considerable trouble remembering what happened in the 30 to 40 minutes prior to the passage of the current.

A somewhat similar behavior has been observed for certain kinds of anesthesia. For example, many patients have trouble remembering what happened just before anesthesia with ether. They can usually remember the mask being put on, but the 30-40 minutes prior to that may be pretty blank.

On this basis, it was generally concluded that, before its final storage, information is in a state where it is easily accessible either for recall or for "erasure." That is, if the patient was either anesthetized or treated with an electroconvulsive shock, the information was not consolidated in the permanent memory and thus must be "forgotten" or erased.

Some experiments with animals seemed consistent with this. Rats were placed in a maze in which they had to make a number of left-right choices in order to get to their reward of a piece of cheese at the other end. These mazes were just complicated enough so that if the rats practiced about 15 minutes each day for a couple of weeks they learned to run with no mistakes. The experimenters then took another group of rats and let them practice for 15 minutes a day, but regularly anesthetized them immediately afterward. These rats just didn't learn. But if the experimenters waited for two hours after the 15-minute session before administering the ether, the rats retained their training and learned almost as rapidly as if they had not been anesthetized at all. As various intervals were tested, again the critical time appeared to be somewhere between 30 and 40 minutes. Thus, when these experiments were reported a number of years ago, we concluded that in man and other animals it must take 40 minutes to store information away permanently.

Then some new experiments were run which caused everyone in this area to sit back and reassess. In this case rats were placed on a wooden pedestal in a fairly large special cage with an electrified floor. Being inquisitive the rats quickly jumped off, and when they hit the floor jumped straight up. While they were in the air, the electricity was turned off, and they were then taken back to their own cages. Whether they were brought back five minutes, an hour, a day, or a year later, they remembered. That is, they would sit on top of their pedestal and quiver and shake, but would not jump off. This is one of the few cases of "one-shot learning" that we know.

The experimenters then tried to erase this information with electroconvulsive shock, by putting electrodes on the ears of the rats so they could pass the surge of current through their brain. However, they could not wait 40 minutes, but rather almost had to catch the rats in the air, for to get any real effect they had to jolt them within 5 to 15 seconds. Many of us who are concerned with this general research area rationalized this by assuming that the length of time information stays in the short-term memory depends upon its urgency.

Some of these original conclusions are apparently correct, whereas others are obviously wrong. For example, a number of recent experiments with animals as well as information available from humans indicate that apparently information is consolidated in the "permanent" memory fairly continuously. But depending upon the circumstances at the time of storage, the information is readily retrievable in some cases, whereas in others it is almost impossible to recall it by normal means. Presumably if the circumstances are pleasant at the time of "permanent consolidation" you put a nice big green flag on it which says, "Recall this whole experience every so often, and you'll be glad you did"; but if consolidation occurs during very unpleasant circumstances, there is a red flag on it which says, "Don't mess around with this—you'll be sorry if you do."

I mention red and green flags because we don't know what physical or chemical features in fact determine retrievability. But we realize that some of our memories can be easily recalled and others only with great difficulty.

EVIDENCE FROM HYPNOSIS AND SURGERY SHOW THAT WE HUMANS HAVE FAR MORE STORED AWAY THAN WE CAN RETRIEVE BY NORMAL PROCEDURES. It now seems fairly evident that not only does information called up under hypnosis represent a true memory recall, but we often also get an undesired bonus. That is, the hypnotized person may embellish the story—apparently in an attempt to please his hypnotizer.

The medical treatment of one defect has provided an unexpected illustration that many experiences are stored away in the permanent memory with a big red flag on them which does not allow us to recall them normally. Older people often get a continual shake of their hand called Parkinsons disease. At least one form of this malady is caused by a malfunction in the thalamus or "switchboard" region deep in the brain. A neurosurgeon dare not go in there with a scalpel, because the damage he would do in passing through the outer layers of the brain would be worse than having the palsy itself. But if an extremely thin electrode (a piece of stiff wire, insulated except at the very end) is put in just the right place, a brief but powerful surge of current can then burn a very minute hole in the thalamus to give a pretty high cure rate for this one type of Parkinsonism. The important point is that the patient must be conscious during the operation so that the clinician knows the electrode is in the right place before he burns the microscopic hole.

During these operations, some surgeons began to stimulate the brain with a weak current, such as is normally found in nerve cells, as they passed the electrode through the outlying layers toward the thalamus, and got quite remarkable results. In some cases the patient would be carrying on a normal conversation with people in the room, but would suddenly "black out" when the electrode was pushed another millimeter; usually they would not come back until it was pushed on still deeper. Sometimes the patients realized that time had passed; in other cases they seemed unaware that anything had happened—in some instances even coming back to the precise place in the sentence where they had broken off.

In one outstanding case, an older woman suddenly began to hum a tune. As luck would have it, in the operating room was a musician who recognized it as being from a certain fairly obscure piece of music. After the operation, he went to the lady's room and began to hum the tune. At first there was no obvious recognition, though this was just a few hours later. When he persisted, however, she finally said, "Oh, I know the name of that piece." She then told him that twenty-three years earlier, while she and her husband were on a vacation at some distance from their home, they came into a small town (which she gave by name), checked into the Grand Hotel at 4:30 in the afternoon, and saw that a classical music program was to be played at 7:30 P.M. at the Roxy Theater. When they arrived at the theater they found it had a bright red door, etc., etc. When the medical personnel checked on her story, they found these and similar details perfectly correct, though both theater and hotel had burned down fifteen years before, so there could have been no recent refreshing of her memory.

There are now about 50 instances on record of this kind of retrieval of information which has been stored away, but which can't be retrieved by normal means. The big question of course is: Will we ever be able to determine exactly where and how to go into the brain to retrieve a particular memory trace or suppress undesired ones? Some experimental operations with epileptics seem to indicate it may be possible, but extremely difficult.

In one form of epilepsy the patient has an aura prior to the seizure. In some cases this involves vivid recall of some scene from the person's past; other patients will hear a piece of music start to play, and when it gets to a certain point in the tune the seizure begins.

Drs. Penfield and Jasper in Montreal put electrodes into the brains of such epileptics, and stimulated with a weak current trying to elicit the aura. Out of the first 1200 patients, they were successful in about 50 cases. In those patients, once the electrode was in proper position, the electrical stimulation "started the music" it played through to the usual specific point, and then the seizure began. If they let the patient recover and did the same thing the next day, they got exactly the same results. When they then burned a microscopic hole at this point, similar to the technique in Parkinsonism, they got "cures" in about a quarter or a third of their patients.

This implies that we can at least initiate the recall of a particular memory event by stimulating a certain place in the brain. Nevertheless, there is other evidence which seems to indicate that all information associated with a given memory trace may not be so highly localized.

WHAT MOTIVATES A PERSON IS ONE OF THE LEAST UNDERSTOOD ASPECTS OF BEHAVIOR. However, the work of Dr. James Olds at the University of Michigan does provide some insight into the most primitive type of motivation. He was interested in determining whether electrical stimulation by electrodes embedded in various parts of a rat's brain would produce unusual specific behavior. A long wire from this electrode was then attached through a switch to a source of electricity so that the rat could stimulate itself by simply pressing the switch.

When certain parts of the brain were stimulated the rat pushed the switch once and only once, and then recoiled as if in great pain. These pain centers were found in various locations in the brain. By contrast, when other regions were stimulated the rat seemed to experience great pleasure, and would stand and push at his switch-bar and forget everything else, such as food, water, or sex. In fact, stimulation of certain pleasure centers seems to give the greatest reward possible for these animals. For instance, if you want to teach an animal to make all the necessary left-right turns to run through a maze, don't put cheese at the other end, but put his switch-bar there and he'll learn in a third to half the time. Furthermore, once a male rat has learned to run through the maze, you can put a female in full heat there and he will pass her by in his eagerness to stimulate his pleasure center. This is the only reward we know that will overwhelm the sex instinct in a male rat—one of the strongest instincts in the animal kingdom.

Moreover, stimulation of a satisfaction center can overcome other potent instincts. For example, an electrode was put into the strongest satisfaction center (which is in the hypothalamus) of a female, and she was then allowed to have a litter of young. A few days later they were put on one side of the cage and she on the other, and separating them was an electrified floor. She refused to go cross that barrier even when her young were molested so that they squealed for help, although she ran up and down indicating her great agitation. But when her switch-bar was put in with her young, she painfully tiptoed across, enduring the shock to her feet in order to get her "kicks."

There are reports that a few prisoners have volunteered for similar tests. And humans do have satisfaction centers which are under better control than in the animals. When the experimenter tells the human to stop pressing the bar, he will, and the experimenter can unplug the apparatus from the wall and from the prisoner's head and leave the room without an actual struggle; whereas the pressing bar can be removed from a rat's cage only with a very heavy glove on because the rat will fight desperately to keep it. With the prisoners, it is found that once they get a look on their face which says they are off on Cloud 9 somewhere, the experimenter can turn off the current and the prisoner will continue to press the bar with the same look of satisfaction. In other words, we know how to initiate satisfaction, but aren't quite sure what is needed to perpetuate it.

In some experiments Olds found that he could get his rats to press for a chemical reward just as avidly as for the electrical reward. In these studies, he inserted a very fine-bore plastic tubing into the brain of the rat rather than an electrode. Now when the rats pushed the switch they would get a microdroplet of chemical. One drop of some chemicals was all they wanted; these presumably are "pain" chemicals. Others seemed to provide just as much pleasure as the electrical stimulus. This suggests that perhaps some chemicals might be used as a reward in manipulating people's behavior, much more efficiently even than electrified floors or the cattle prod.

WHAT SHOULD WE DO WITH THESE TECHNIQUES? There are many cases of human memory in which, if it were possible, we would be glad to change green flags to red. As an illustration, you probably read with horror during the Christmas season a few years ago about the policeman's teen-age daughter who was selling Christmas cards or candy in Los Angeles and was dragged into a house and raped repeatedly by a bunch of thugs. As a consequence she reverted to the behavior of an eight- or ten-year-old child with severe mental depression and retardation, though excellent psychiatrists tried unsuccessfully to treat her. They simply were not able to rescue her because they could not blot out her memory of horror.

How wonderful it would be if we could put a red flag on the happenings of that day and restore her to a normal, productive life. But who determines what things we should suppress with red flags? (Certainly if we begin doing this there are a few *little* things I have said during my married life which I would love to have my wife forget.)

Alternatively, changing red flags to green could be of tremendous benefit in certain kinds of psychotherapy. Initially, many of us had hoped LSD would provide a means of getting information out deliberately, easily, and without injury, since it seemed to cause a tremendous increase in people's awareness of their senses and perhaps also of past happenings. However, LSD appears to produce a tremendous number of bad side effects—in particular, chromosome aberrations leading to seriously defective offspring.

It is to be hoped that we may be able to adapt some of our new knowledge on how the mind functions so as to develop the tools needed to transform a Caryl Chessman or others with various mental disorders. For example, Caryl Chessman spent twelve or thirteen years on death row in California and wrote an impressive book, which indicated quite an outstanding intellect. But, tragically, he also liked to rape girls and kill their boyfriends in lover's lane. If we had been able to go in and change some values in that brain, we might have retrieved a worthy member for society.

But the question is, if we can learn how to erase and rewrite, *who decides* what values are to go into the mind that is being manipulated?

Should it be a Chessman? After all he is largely responsible for getting himself into his trouble.

Should it be the psychiatrist? Most psychiatrists believe they should get a patient to understand why he is misbehaving, rather than decide themselves what kind of a person that patient ought to be. In fact, one of the reasons for only limited advancement in this area of mind manipulation is that we scientists simply do not know what rights and obligations we have, even for doing the research to develop these techniques.

Should society decide what Chessman should be like? In Orwell's book *1984*, Big Brother government decided what everyone should think.

Or should the parents be involved? Yet they may have been an important factor in creating the problem.

But I have dwelt on Caryl Chessman really to set the stage for a more important question. Let us now disregard both Chessman and the unusual situation he represents.

WOULD YOU SAY THAT PARENTS SHOULD BE PRIMARILY RESPONSIBLE FOR THE VALUES OF THEIR CHILDREN? If like most people you say, yes, then the far more critical question comes next. Let's suppose we can develop mind manipulation techniques to the point where parents can put the desired values into their children pretty much as we would program a computer. Would you want to use this technique?

I am always surprised, in lecturing, when most people vote yes on the first question, but I don't see any hands raised on this last question. This says that most people are voting that parents *are* supposed to be responsible for the values of their children—but should not be deliberate about it. That's nothing but sloppy parent-hood! Although you may smile, I'm sure you get the point!

What *are* our obligations, once we bring a child into this world? How deliberate should we be about instilling in him a definite set of values? Many of our problems today—e.g. in hippieland—exist because parents have been unwilling or unable to assume this re-sponsibility. All too often people seem to think that just procreating a life is all there is to parenthood. Nothing could be further from the truth. Two fools in a drunken stupor can bring a child into this world. No—suddenly that little child arrives, unable to do any-thing, and if it doesn't get values we know what is going to happen. This means we must play God for that child by giving it a set of values, if we are going to do a proper job of being parents. But although this is our obligation as individual parents, do we have a further obligation as a society?

HOW DELIBERATE SHOULD WE BE IN GIVING VALUES TO THOSE YOUNGSTERS WHOSE PARENTS DON'T PROVIDE THEM WITH AN ADEQUATE SET? This is one of the most crucial, brutal questions facing us today. Such youngsters are found throughout society; in fact, the highest percentage increase in crime today is found among the young people in our affluent suburbs. Nevertheless, we must be most concerned about the problem in our inner-city ghettoes.

I first became aware of what can happen to youngsters in the ghetto when I was at the University of Chicago in 1949 and 1950, just when the south side of the city was in a tremendous state of flux. Six of my fellow students and I lived on the third floor of an apartment building in what we thought were quite crowded condi-tions. But on the floor below was a group supported by ADC (Aid to Dependent Children). Grandma had moved in with her three daughters and their offspring—*twenty-three* of them in the same space as we seven occupied. I got to know the oldest male member of that household fairly well—young George was seven years old. He was spawned because the very fine ADC program had been thwarted and warped by his mother. She had learned that the break-even point for board, room, and liquor was five kids, and George was the second in line. Unfortunately, to his mother he represented a certain number of dollars each month. He was put out in the morning, sat on the front stoop, and was let back in at night. That front stoop was his station in life.

Another white student and I were the only semblance of a father this Negro lad had ever had, for we were the only males who ever stopped to talk to him. It was quite an experience to try to tell or read to little George about Snow White and the Seven Dwarfs or Jack and the Beanstalk because George had never seen a book. You knew full well that he did not have much of any place to go in this world.

When I campaigned for the State Board of Education in Michigan in the fall of 1966, it was brought forcefully home to me once again that unfortunately, little George is not unique. I recall vividly the day I went into a counselor's office in one of the ghetto high schools and found him very dejected. He said, "I think I probably have sentenced three young men to jail. Although they weren't misbehaving too badly, I had to kick them out of school because otherwise discipline in the whole school would have disintegrated. The problem is, they have nowhere to go." He went on, "When you are done campaigning tonight you come around, and I'll show you what I mean." And so about eleven thirty that evening we entered a dilapidated "apartment house" and walked down the hall to the very narrow door of a janitor's closet. My friend opened it slowly, and there, standing upright in one corner, leaning back slightly and fast asleep, was one of these young men. It was a warm spot.

We walked a block and a half down the street to an even worse place, and there under the stairway was the second boy. The family across the hallway was good enough to let him use their bathroom each morning. He owned exactly two pairs of pants, three shirts and one complete change of underwear.

"Why doesn't this boy go home?" I said.

The counselor snorted. "He doesn't know what you are talking about when you use that word. He never knew who his father was, and when he was eight his mother left him with the neighbors while she went shopping. A few days later an envelope came with twenty-five dollars in it, and a letter that said, 'Joe and I have gone to Arizona. When we strike it rich we'll send for you.' He was eight then. He is sixteen now. Apparently they haven't struck it rich yet."

This was before the riots of 1967, and even then it was estimated there were 8,000 to 10,000 such youngsters in the city of Detroit who did not have a home. Detroit is not unique; the McCone report describing the riot in Los Angeles points out that the rioters in Watts were a remarkably homogeneous group of fellows between the ages of fourteen and twenty-two. When they were picked up, they would say their name was Joe. But when they were asked, "Joe what?" invariably they said, "I don't know." Initially, the police thought they were just trying to escape detection; then they began to find out that they simply didn't know who they were—like our second young man, they had never known who their father was, and their mothers often put them out on the streets from the age of eight or ten on. In fact, out of 336 households in one of the largest housing developments in Watts, only 11 had a resident father.

Why don't these youngsters behave like those of us in the middle class? Need we ask? In fact, it was surprising that during the riots so many people should exclaim, "What do they hope to gain from burning down the cities?" For one of these youngsters it's the wrong question. Their feeling is, "What do I have to lose?" And if we were in their place our attitude would probably be the same.

Another factor contributing to the deficiencies of these youngsters is the kind of education available in the ghetto. In the report of the Civil Rights Commission to the President entitled *The Racial Isolation in Our Public Schools* we get the following picture. Suppose two children live on opposite sides of a street that divides two school districts. If one youngster goes to an essentially all-Negro school for twelve years, his average achievement will be at the seventh- to ninth-grade level. However, this doesn't mean these youngsters are deficient in basic mental capacity because if his friend goes for twelve years to a predominantly white school, his average achievement will be at the eleventh- or twelfth-grade level. One boy who had attended both types of schools emphasized an important contrast between the two, the goals held up before the students. "In the suburbs they asked me which college I was going to attend, whereas in the city they talked about whether I would make it through high school."

With this background the obvious question is: *What do we do about it—what kind of action do we need?* Many of these youngsters will go nowhere unless we give them a set of values.

One place to attack this lack of values (at least by the standards of the rest of society) is in a program like Operation Headstart. In this program, youngsters three to five years old are brought in to learn some words and concepts so that they can cope with school when they finally get into the first grade. The program is badly needed, for many of these youngsters have a vocabulary of barely 400 or 500 words at this age.

This brings me to another story I simply have not been able to get out of my mind. One of our student teachers from Michigan State University who was helping in an Operation Headstart program showed her youngsters pictures of toys you would find in most middle-class families. When she held up a picture of a teddy bear none of the ten youngsters in the class could identify it. Finally one little four-year-old girl said hesitantly, "Is it a rat?"

To a certain extent Operation Headstart is helping to correct these deficiencies. But as the people in the program will tell you, its real success is that somebody takes one of these youngsters and sets him on their knee and says in effect, "Look, little George—it's important to me that you are little George." Very possibly no one has ever made this youngster feel that before!

NOW COMES THE BRUTAL QUESTION. DO WE GO ONE CRITICAL STEP FURTHER AND CHANGE THAT GHETTO CHILD'S VALUES? As I, too, found from personal experience, once young George is convinced that somebody does care, suddenly that little mind opens up, and it is a blank slate on which we can write. Accordingly, should the person on whose knee he sits in an Operation Headstart or similar program go the next step further and say, "Incidentally, if you want to get along in this world, little George, you had better adopt my middle-class set of values"—?

If you say, "Oh no, we don't ever have the right to determine a set of values for someone else, and especially for someone else's child," then you have just consigned that youngster to society's scrapheap. For unless we change the whole fabric of our society, that young person cannot compete in life without an adequate set of values.

If you say, "Yes, we have an obligation to give these youngsters a set of values, so that they can compete!," then I must ask one further question: *Whose* values? Frankly, I am surprised always in speaking to audiences to find that more than 50 per cent of those asked—black and white alike—usually say we have an obligation to give the ghetto youngsters a set of values; yet almost no one raises a hand to say that they should be deliberate about putting values into their own children. Can anyone who doesn't have the guts to be deliberately responsible for the values of his own children *ever* presume to specify values for someone else's?

I believe we really have no choice but to provide these youngsters with a set of values. In fact, this year I commuted ninety miles to Detroit on Saturday mornings, trying to brainwash some seniors in one of the ghetto high schools into believing both that it is good to go on to college and that they can make it if they are willing to try. I taught them material which I have given as a freshman course at the University, so that they could see what would be expected of them if they came to college. This attempt to break down their "creditability gap" is essential, for last year this school graduated only slightly more than 250 seniors—the residue from about 1000 sophomores and (as nearly as we can tell) about 1500 youngsters at the sixth-grade level. Fewer than 30 of them went on to college, and only 2 or 3 of these stand a reasonable chance of making it through their first year. Probably most people approve of my effort; however, if I began to try and sell some other values in which I believe equally strongly, there might not be such good agreement.

Since this brutal choice cannot be disregarded if our society is to hold together, we dare not say this is somebody else's problem. Values will be put in by those who commute to the ghetto high schools on Saturday mornings, or by those who provide an understanding knee for the little Georges who participate in Operation Headstart. Of particular importance, such programs may eventually involve 10 to 15 per cent of our population. Thus I repeat: if you are unwilling to deliberately put values into your own children, can you possibly presume to participate in a decision as to what should go into someone else's children?

There is a third alternative to the brutal alternatives I have posed. That is, to change the whole fabric of our society to accommodate the different values which we find in some of our ghetto people. Although I believe very strongly in most of the fundamental principles—though not always the operating procedures—of my middle-class society, ghetto people have many virtues also. One of these is a lack of hypocrisy which is all too often not found in my own class. Wherever possible, all of us must insist that values be put into youngsters in such a way there can be a real give-and-take between those who would give and those who receive.

In this connection my wife Elizabeth and I initiated Operation Get-Acquainted in our home community last year.* Under this program Negro ADC youngsters were guests in white middle-class homes for a week or ten days during the summer. We were trying to get together the two groups who must assume critical roles in resolving one of today's most worrisome problems: the Negro youngster who must kick open the door of opportunity, and the white middle class which controls our society and thus the lock on that door. One of the outstanding virtues of this program is that here youngsters are exposed to a different way of life, or values, or whatever term we may want to use, in a situation where both sides have a chance to observe each other's good and bad qualities. The fact is, I hope my Davey will grow up to be as respectful of his parents as was our little 8-year-old guest, Erwin. The latter certainly had some very endearing qualities, and also some others that I would like to see changed. Whether he adopts our values or not, of course, remains his future choice. And I learned from him and 12-year-old Valerie, who also visited us, that they have both strengths and weaknesses. As a member of the Michigan State Board of Education, I now have a better idea what we must deal with in trying to design programs to help these youngsters. This is the kind of give and take we must have.

Clearly, this is an area in which we must all be concerned. The

*Although we thought Operation Get-Acquainted was brand new we found later that it mimics very closely the Fresh Air Fund and Friendly Town programs which have been operating in 12 Eastern States for years.

techniques are highly advanced for manipulating behavior without caring what goes on internally. In addition, even though we in science cannot at the moment explain how brainwashing works, techniques are available right now for at least limited mind manipulation. If our society decides that we need these techniques very much, probably a number of laboratories will begin to work quite hard on further development. The big question is, are we ready to use this information and these techniques?

In the ghetto, as everyone knows, we face the brutal choice mentioned above. But in reality that same hard choice is found wherever we consider putting these techniques to use. The alternatives are awesome; we dare not delay in facing the decisions that must be made. By the same token, we dare not be hasty or unmindful of the consequences. Because, you see, the mind is a refuge and a fortress for many things.

If we use our newfound capabilities properly, we can attack and destroy the final sanctuary of inequality, ignorance, and incompetence. By the same token, if we misuse these techniques, we will undoubtedly attack and destroy the last stronghold of integrity and individualism.

"I'll be judge, I'll be the jury," said cunning old Fury:
"I'll try the whole cause, and condemn you to death."
—*Alice in Wonderland*

✷

CHAPTER 7

Button, Button, Who Has the Button?*

As the new crucial, complex decisions confront us, we must ask not only *What is the right thing to do?* and *What set of values do we use?* but also *Who should be making the decisions?* In fact, very often the decision as to who will decide also determines what set of values will come into play. Unfortunately, we are ill-prepared at the moment to make these determinations, whether at the federal, local, or individual level. As a consequence, in many real-life situations adults essentially play the old children's game of "Button, button, who's got the button?" as they search frantically—and often tragically—for the proper person or group to assume responsibility.

THE INADEQUACIES AT THE FEDERAL LEVEL ARE WELL RE-VEALED BY TWO ILLUSTRATIONS. For over two years, applications for licensing two different drugs submitted by two different companies have been lying on the desk of a friend of mine who serves in the Food and Drug Administration. Both drugs have been very

---

*The general question of "Who shall decide?" was first discussed publicly in the form presented here while I was campaigning in Michigan for the Republican nomination for the U. S. Senate in 1966.

effective in combating leukemia in laboratory animals. Unfortunately, though, both drugs appear to work because they produce large numbers of mutations, some of which have severe repercussions: these include blindness, inability to digest many kinds of food, periodic seizures, and so on. Of greatest consequence, many of these defects are passed on to the next generation.

Clearly these applications for testing in humans should be given careful scrutiny. If you license them for use in women of fifty or over who are not going to have children, then I personally don't have a moral question mark. It should be their choice whether they want to live but take a chance on being moderately or even severely uncomfortable. It is quite a different problem, though, if you license them for testing in women of forty or below, or in males of any age up to sixty or seventy, who can potentially still procreate a child.

Who should make this decision? Some people argue that it should not be someone in the Food and Drug Administration, since my friend is about eight layers deep in the federal bureaucracy, and thus if you don't like what he does there really isn't anything you can do to change his decision. This is not to say that my friend is unethical or insensitive at all; he is quite the opposite. However—since he and his colleagues are not directly accountable to the electorate—some people say, let's not have the FDA bottling up these and similar drug applications, but pass the decision on to the individuals involved. Specifically, if an adult is treated, let that person decide whether he or she will take the chance of passing on a serious mutation to the next generation, or will take some measure(s) not to have any children.

Then comes the problem, what about children? Some argue that it is the obligation of the parents to make the decision. However, if one of my children develops leukemia at the age of six or eight, if there is any drug around which will save Davey's or Kim's life, then Elizabeth and I will see to it that they are treated. I certainly won't be concerned about the grandchildren at that point. Some go a step further and say, let the parents save the life of the child, but then the child should decide what it is going to do when it gets to a responsible age. This now means that at the age of twelve or thirteen I must tell Davey or Kim, "Incidentally, I saved your life back there when you were seven, but now you are a hazard to the next generation. Since you will soon be able to procreate a life, you should consider having yourself sterilized to make absolutely sure you are not responsible for imposing a real catastrophe on your children—my grandchildren." It is hardly being realistic to expect a child to make such a catastrophic decision just when he is struggling to establish his own self-identity.

Still other people believe that the decision should be made by the doctor together with the individuals involved. That is, they argue that the FDA should determine the potentialities and also the dangers of a given drug and then make sure that all doctors know all the details. There are obvious virtues in this mode of proceeding, but there are also serious disadvantages. There are now not just one or two but a large number of drugs which no longer affect simply the individual receiving the drug but also have consequences for their offspring. Thus, with more and more occasions arising, will the individuals involved, or the doctors plus the individuals involved, always provide adequate protection for that next generation?

During a discussion on one of my TV shows the dilemma was very well put by one of my guests. I had deliberately put my visitors on the spot by asking them whether anyone receiving such a drug should have to be sterilized first, so as to protect the next generation. Somewhat surprisingly, the youngest unmarried person on the panel, who would have the most to lose, immediately said yes, he thought that "Whoever had a mutation produced by such a treatment would be like a live time bomb walking around in our society. We don't allow someone with diphtheria or some other dread infectious disease to go around endangering the public, so why should we create such a danger to the next generation and then not give them the same kind of protection we provide for people already here?" Almost unanimously the older members of the group discussing the problem jumped in and pointed out that this was analogous to Hitler's rationale. While our fears may be justified, the young man's reasoning cannot be disregarded, nor can the question be avoided: Who should decide this matter?

We have not really had this question in the past, simply because most drugs produced an effect only on the person taking them. Thus the function of the FDA has been mainly to insure that drugs are both "effective"—that is, they do what their label claims—and "safe." Obviously, if a drug is effective in combating one disease but kills a patient for another reason, this is not a very good bargain. But how do we define the term, "safe" when the next generation may be involved? Thalidomide was effective in combating some of the early problems encountered in pregnancy, and it did not cause any undesirable side effects in a woman herself. However, it surely clobbered some children.

No matter who makes the decision, initially it has to be made on the basis of inadequate knowledge. The problem is quite simple. Even with extensive data on laboratory animals, we still cannot be sure that we will not get a serious side effect until we have actually tested many of the new drugs in man. Thus, if we do not license a drug for testing so long as there is a *chance* that it may cause serious side effects in humans or their offspring, then almost no new drugs can be put on the market. I am not in favor of that, if my child is suffering from leukemia.

THE AUTHORIZATION OF RESEARCH ON GENE MANIPULATION WILL POSE SIMILAR NATIONAL PROBLEMS IN TESTING. I have already discussed in Chapter 2 the tricky questions and risks associated with viruses which might be used for manipulating defective genes. As with the drugs discussed above, we can test these preparations and methods in two or ten or twenty different types of laboratory animals without any serious side effects, yet never be sure that there are no consequences for man himself until we have tested them in humans, because we are not genetically identical with any other animal.

There are rumors that at least two laboratories will submit requests soon to the federal government for funds to seek out viruses to manipulate additional defective genes. The decision to give or not to give money for the proposed research will be made by scientific specialists at the National Institutes of Health, the National Science Foundation, or some similar funding agency. I have served in this capacity with both the Atomic Energy Commission and the National Institutes of Health. Although the exact procedures differ from agency to agency, in most cases decisions are made by a panel of anywhere from five to twelve scientists. When I served on a panel for dealing with drugs that affect nerve and brain functioning, we got a few "noncontroversial" requests for research on drugs such as LSD, etc. When these came up, invariably there was a discussion not only of the scientific merit of the proposal, but also of the ethical considerations involved. Eventually someone would say, Look, we're not a bunch of ministers, we're here to carry out our mandate of deciding whether these people can do the science which they propose.

If these two research proposals on gene manipulation are evaluated strictly on scientific merit and potential, then they certainly will be funded, because they will be submitted by absolutely top-notch scientists. Yet, whether it be licensing of leukemia drugs, authorizing research on a virus to be used in humans, or authorizing and funding research on mind manipulation, the decision cannot rest simply on an evaluation of scientific elegance, efficiency, or sophistication.

Furthermore, our elected representatives are not directly involved in such earth-shaking decisions either. Congress cannot possibly look at each $250,000 item!

But this is not just any old $250,000 item! If such research is funded, and if it is successful in turning up some promising viruses —or other materials or methods—for manipulating genes, then the next critical decision will be made when the FDA must decide whether to license the material for testing in humans. This is the problem discussed above. The final critical administrative move is made when the FDA decides whether or not the material is to be put on the open market for widespread clinical use.

To further illustrate the kind of pitfalls we can stumble into: suppose we were to find a virus which carried the necessary DNA for correcting diabetes and made all the boys very tall (good basketball teams) and raised their IQ's by fifteen points (no flunking out of school). If any laboratory announced such a virus, the pressures to license it both for testing and for widespread use would be just unbelievable, since it is estimated that at least one out of every five persons has at least one defective gene for diabetes. Suppose though, we were unlucky and the virus contained not only a certain amount of DNA, enabling people to make their own insulin, but additional DNA so that the group tested either went on to have defective children or developed schizophrenia. We would have a whole generation with extensive genetic changes *before we even knew they were in trouble.*

Who should decide? How cautiously should we or, in fact, could we move? And on and on go the questions.

To summarize, there are really only five places where the critical decision of "go or no-go" can be made. The *first* place is in the mind of the scientist who gets the initial idea. But if he decides not to proceed because the possible repercussions are too great, he then really plays God in denying any possible help to future children who may develop leukemia, and so on. The *second* place is in the scientific funding groups. Unfortunately, these groups are not directly responsible to the electorate.

The *third* and *fourth* places are at the Food and Drug Administration, at the time a drug is licensed either for testing or later for general distribution. The *final* place where decisions can be made is in a public controversy such as we had with nuclear testing.

The conflict over nuclear testing certainly exemplifies the problems that arise when decisions are made without the direct and formal involvement of the three kinds of people who should contribute to these kinds of decisions: the scientist, with his knowledge of how things work and what is possible technically; the person from the humanities, with his set of values; and the politician, with his expertise in how to get things done. No one of these three groups is more or less important than the other, and no one group can do the job by itself.

OUR DECISION-MAKING APPARATUS MUST BE REVAMPED to make sure that these groups are brought together in a formal way when critical decisions are made. Accordingly, I recently proposed the following procedure.

In existing practice, when any scientist submits a proposal for research funds which involves the use of either humans or animals, we must submit a statement that the experiments will be carried out with proper safeguards for their well-being. This must be further certified by a university (or industry) committee which has formal obligations to insure that humane procedures are followed. Similar assurances of safe procedures must be given if we employ radioactive isotopes in our research. Further, in his progress reports the scientist must include a statement as to whether he has or has not made patentable discoveries or developments while utilizing federal funds.

I have therefore proposed that we now do the same sort of thing concerning the possible ethical implications and consequences if a given piece of research is successful. Such a statement, contained in the funding proposal and also buttressed by an independent evaluation from a group of scientists and humanists at the university level, could then be forwarded to the group responsible for authorizing and funding research within the national agencies. If the group in the National Institutes of Health, or the Atomic Energy Commission, etc., had not only scientists but also some people from the humanities on their panel, they could then recommend how to control the developments of any procedures or products that might arise from the research proposed. In particular, this group should now have the obligation to make sure that Congress knows the possible implications of research being considered.

Finally, I have proposed the establishment of a statutory group to advise Congress on these matters. This group, of course, is the one which would bring together in a formal way the scientists, the humanists, and the politicians. At the moment the only statutory science advisory group we have at the federal level is responsible only to the executive branch; Congress does not have such advice available except in crisis situations, when they hold hearings on some matter or other.

My proposal is that we scientists (and also those in the humanities) elect some of our colleagues to positions on this statutory advisory group to Congress. I feel very strongly that those who either are engaged in, or have the potential for, making profound changes in our society should be not only represented but, more importantly, held accountable. At the moment the group of scientists advising the executive branch are all advisers without porfolio, and I think in the long run this is not a healthy situation.

Certainly we must avoid the temptation to assign—either deliberately or by default—the developments and decisions in these areas to a single agency, as happened with nuclear testing. By statute the Atomic Energy Commission was directed to determine the problems in the area of nuclear energy, to secure funds from

Congress to do needed research, to authorize and administer the research, to analyze and evaluate the experimental results in this area, and to refine and revamp the problems associated with nuclear energy. That is, the AEC was set up by law to be "judge, jury, and executioner." Fortunately, I know from working at the AEC that most of their many employees have been concerned and committed persons. Moreover, I agree with most of the major decisions made by this agency. Nevertheless, I feel this would be a basically unhealthy, if not downright dangerous, arrangement for the decisions now confronting us.

Those who know me well, I am sure, are surprised that I would ever recommend establishing such a potentially unwieldy arrangement, because I so deplore bureaucracy and involved committee structures. Certainly I recognize that my proposed changes would increase the red tape associated with my own work. However, the issues are so crucial and the stakes so great that I believe this price must be paid to insure that the decision makers are directly responsible to those they represent!

THE DEFICIENCIES IN THE DECISION-MAKING APPARATUS AT THE LOCAL LEVEL ARE COMPARABLE TO THOSE AT THE FEDERAL LEVEL. Decisions about the operation of kidney machines can illustrate the inadequacy very vividly.

There are new machines in many communities around the country which can be used to clean up a person's blood stream when their kidneys go bad. Unfortunately, the supply of machines is inadequate for the number of people who need them. In most communities the time requested exceeds the time available by a factor of anywhere from 5:1 to 30:1. Someone must decide who are to be the "lucky ones" who get on the machine; but more importantly, they have to decide who doesn't. For when a decision is made not to let someone on a machine, then the deciders have just signed the unlucky patient's death warrant, merely leaving the day and hour blank. Some people might argue that with our affluence this should never be a problem—that we should simply build enough machines to service everyone. Even assuming we could find all the trained people to service the machines, it would still cost about $2 billion a year to take care of the 10,000 or so individuals who need a machine. This is approximately the amount spent by the federal government (through the National Institutes of Health) for research on *all types* of medical problems. Thus the need to choose among a number of kidney patients is going to be with us for quite a while, unless overnight somebody invents a simpler machine which can supplant those now in use.

In some hospitals the doctors alone choose those to be treated on their kidney machine. At others it is the doctors plus hospital administrators who decide. In a very few communities it is a panel of citizens-at-large who assume this burden.

I talked recently to a man and woman who serve on such a jury, and they described the difficulties encountered in one of their decisions. A block of time had become available on the machine for which they were responsible. There were 11 applicants, all of whom the doctors said would profit from the treatment. After much deliberation they narrowed the choice down to three people. Let me describe the finalists.

The first was a well-known, productive sixty-two-year old author. He has had not only a family of fine children, but now grandchildren. By any standards he has lived a full life. However, he is now writing a novel in which he is trying to depict the forces at work on a youngster in the ghetto. And this panel of busy people took time out to read the first three chapters in draft form. It was their evaluation that if he could carry on at the same level for the rest of the book it would be of tremendous value to those of us in the middle class who are trying to understand what we can best do to help youngsters in the ghetto. Probably he could finish the book in two years or less, and they could keep him alive for that long. If he were the choice then society would benefit.

The second of this trio was a woman in her middle fifties with three teen-age daughters at home. However, she was an alcoholic trying to take the cure for the third time. Selecting her would give her a chance to recover a wholesome life and look after her youngsters at home.

The third finalist was a thirty-seven-year-old manager of a loan company with three children (one, two, and seven years old) at home. Even though he was voted the ousstanding young man of the year in his community two years ago, he had just deserted his family. But the panel was fairly certain that he had done this in order not to be a burden on them.

Whom would you choose? The author? The mother? The young man? And again, who should make this choice? Some people will argue that a computer should decide this sort of thing, since it would be impartial and not subject to human vagaries. In fact, there is one great virtue in having any choice made by a computer: at least you know all the factors that went into the decision. But can we decide which of three people should get onto a kidney machine in a purely cold-blooded, analytical way? This citizens' panel had an interesting rule. If any member of the jury knew one of the applicants personally, he (or she) was obligated to disqualify himself (herself). The argument that this would be unfair to other applicants is obvious. On the other hand, is it really possible to choose among the three people listed without knowing them as individuals? Yet again, any married man knows quite well that even though he has lived with his wife for twenty years, still she will continually surprise him. Could any jury ever get to know applicants well enough so as to determine their "worth" as an individual?

THE RIGHTS AND OBLIGATIONS OF THE INDIVIDUAL AND SOCIETY ARE ALSO DIFFICULT TO DETERMINE UNEQUIVOCALLY IN MANY INSTANCES. One of the most tragic cases in which I have participated arose because there were no clearcut guidelines as to who should really be responsible. My involvement came about as follows.

I received a long-distance phone call from a couple whose first mongoloid child had died in the first year of life. Then followed two normal children, and their fourth child was another mongoloid. The mother was now pregnant and they wanted to know what the chances were that their fifth child would again be defective. Accordingly, I made arrangements with their doctor for chromosome tests to be run on the living mongoloid child. These showed that this was a translocation or "piggy-back" mongoloid (see Chapter 2), which meant that the chances for the fetus the mother was now carrying to be defective ranged from approximately one out of six to one out of three. When the parents heard this, they asked for tests to determine whether they had hit the one-out-of-three probability that the child would be defective or the two-out-of-three probability it would be normal. Arrangements were made for the tests on cells taken from the amniotic fluid and in the fifth month of pregnancy I heard that this fetus was another mongoloid.

Then the complications began. Although the doctor had made all the arrangements for the previous tests, he now abruptly decided he would not pass on the information to the parents, because he was sure from their religious beliefs they would insist upon an abortion. They happened to be Congregationalists who did not have the same taboos as he himself did, being a fairly conservative Catholic.

I argued with him off and on for approximately two weeks that the information should be passed on to the parents so that they could make their own decision. When I was unsuccessful, I passed the results on to the minister who had also counseled and advised this couple. We debated off and on for the next few weeks whether we should tell the parents. Although we did not like this long delay (for the mother was now entering the seventh month), both the minister and I were reluctant to assume individual responsibility for destroying the doctor-patient relationship between this couple and their doctor who were also very close personal friends. He had continued to tell them that the tests were inconclusive, and in fact had even acted out the subterfuge of removing additional amniotic fluid for a fictitious retest. Finally we decided that it was our obligation to let the parents know, and accordingly, a meeting was arranged at their home for the next Saturday.

When I arrived I was instructed by the oldest boy to go directly to the hospital because "Momma is going to have a baby." In the hospital waiting room I came into one of the most explosive situations I have ever encountered. The doctor, the father, and the minister were in urgent argument about what should be done. The mother had indeed gone into labor—very abnormal labor. The doctor's prognosis was that if the labor were allowed to continue for even half an hour, very likely the fetus would be killed, but the mother's life could be saved by an operation. However, both the baby's and mother's lives could be saved by an immediate Caesarean. After a two-minute briefing I was asked for my advice. I told the father, who now knew that this child was a mongoloid, what I would do in such a situation. About this time the nurse came to the door and indicated to the doctor that the fetal heartbeat had slowed quite appreciably, and the doctor said he had to have an immediate decision. The father stood shifting his weight from one foot to the other and arguing out loud with himself, until abruptly the doctor said, "If you can't make up your mind, John, I am going to do what my conscience tells me I should." He immediately left to perform the Caesarean.

A few minutes later I pointed out to the father that he must now face still another decision. I knew personally of two cases where a mother was presented with her third grossly defective child and simply could not stand the shock—in fact, it would take either an unbelievably strong or unbelievably callous individual not to be greatly affected by such an occurrence. One alternative would be to do what I had heard about in another somewhat comparable situation; namely, to have a false stillborn birth certificate issued for the benefit of the mother, and then to put the child in an institution. If much later—when the mother was past the post-birth blues, etc. —the father and other competent persons decided that she could take the shock, she could be told the truth and they could decide what should be done with the child at that point. Alternatively, if he was still undecided what to do, he could buy time for making his own decision by telling the mother that since it was a premature birth it was uncertain whether the child would live, and they could keep it in an incubator until they decided.

Both the minister and I urged as strongly as we could that the father employ the phony stillborn birth certificate, since this would buy the maximum amount of time to decide. The husband seemed to agree and requested that I ask the doctor's advice. The latter not only agreed that this was a wise procedure, but gave me the name of a judge he thought might be sympathetic and willing to issue the false certificate, keeping the real one sealed in his records. I tried to call the judge, but he was out of town for the weekend.

When I returned to the waiting room, the minister was just finishing a prayer asking for guidance. I told the father about the doctor's comments and also that the judge could not be reached immediately. There were a few minutes of dead silence, after which the father suddenly blurted out, "I won't be responsible for making this decision. My wife and I have come through our trials and tribulations together up until now. We will tell her about the child and together she and I will decide what to do." Both the minister and I argued strongly against this course, and in a few minutes we were joined by the doctor. But it became obvious that the husband had made up his mind and was becoming more and more intractable and finally almost irrational. The doctor delayed matters by saying that the mother had not yet recovered from the operation and that the child needed special care. As the father became more and more aggressive, we considered having him removed forcibly from the hospital and put under temporary sedation.

For better or worse, this idea was finally abandoned, and about six hours after the operation the very distraught husband was allowed to see his wife. When he blurted out what had happened, she almost immediately went into shock, but by the next day seemed to recover fairly well. However, during her recuperation, the child had to be rescued from her when she tried to kill it. At this point she became more and more violent and uncontrollable, and is now in a padded cell under constant guard because she tries continually to defeminize herself.

My initial reaction was utter contempt for this weak-kneed father. But I have had to make mental apologies to him many times over, for within a week after the commitment of his wife, he pulled himself together from his own severe shock, put both mongoloid children into an institution, and is now building a strong home life for the other two. I do not think the man was any more irresponsible than the rest of us would have been, had we found ourselves unexpectedly in a similarly urgent and difficult situation.

I blamed myself bitterly, and also the minister, for not deciding earlier that the parents must be informed. However, I can salve our consciences by pointing out that we had no *real* responsibility. We were involved in the case only by invitation. And I have often condemned the doctor for denying the information to his patients. Yet, by the same token, if he had passed it on I am sure these very close friends of his would have brought unbearable pressure to bear on him, either to terminate that life himself, or at least to make arrangements with some colleague to do the abortion. Given his background and beliefs, I am not sure I could have done anything very different.

The real culprit is the system—or more accurately, the lack of a system—for making these decisions. Who do you think should have decided in this case? The doctor? The parents? Society (which the minister and I represented informally)? In our culture today we have not determined who should make these decisions. And this is a luxury·we can no longer afford.

People pay a high price with their shattered lives when critical decisions are not made or when the individuals are not strong enough to face the consequences. Thus, we must consider still another facet of this general question of *Who shall decide?*

SHOULD EITHER INDIVIDUALS OR SOCIETY PROVIDE A CRUTCH TO PEOPLE FACING ALMOST SUPERHUMAN DECISIONS? The dilemma of the young man involved in the grandson-to-grandfather kidney transplant provides still' another illustration of how critical this whole phase of human deciding can be. When I first talked to the grandfather, he said quite bluntly, "As a surgeon I have been making this kind of decision for family after family, week after week, year after year, for over forty years. It's somebody else's turn to make one for me. I didn't ask for the kidney, but if it is given to me, I will operate day and night as long as I can." No one could really fault him for this attitude, and so this left it squarely up to the grandson.

After about two weeks of wrestling with their problem, I realized that the grandson was going to get hurt no matter what he did. Even if his grandfather received the kidney, operated for five full years, and saved a thousand lives—ten years later, if the grandson's other kidney goes bad, he cannot look his two children, now ten and twelve years old, in the eye and say that he had their best interests at heart when he became a donor. By the same token, if the grandson did not go through with it, he would no doubt feel guilty when his grandfather died—but think what would happen as he read the obituary lists during the next few years in that community and realized that person after person was dying who could have been saved if his grandfather had been there to operate.

About three weeks after I was contacted, I received a call that the grandfather was going in and out of a coma and that they would have to operate within a couple of days or forget about it. I made arrangements for the grandson to call three different researchers so as to evaluate the deficit in his life expectancy if he went ahead. While he talked with the third one, I listened in on a conference-call arrangement and found that he was really trying hard to justify giving the kidney rather than trying to find some way to "chicken out."

Accordingly, when the conversation was over, I advised him to go through with the operation since he would be placed at the top of the priority list for a kidney machine if he needed it in the future. Secondly, arrangements had been made for the grandfather to carry a rather unusual set of identification, so that if he were involved in an accident or were to have a heart attack, the attending physician's first consideration would be to retrieve the kidney and give it back to the grandson. (This raises a bizarre but genuine side issue: suppose the operation is carried out and the grandson's other kidney goes bad while the grandfather is still alive. Who should have the preeminent right to the first kidney? The grandfather? The grandson?)

The fact was that on another sheet of paper I had equally persuasive arguments against the donation. I was trying to convince him that I had in fact made the decision for him. Was this a favor to him or not? Certainly if he can make this decision and then live with the consequences later on, he will achieve a maturity that cannot be achieved really in any other way. By the same token, if something goes wrong, how many people do you know who can be expected to survive the consequences without severe repercussions? We have only to think back to the father suddenly faced with the birth of his third mongoloid child, or the sensitive wife in a Puerto Rico hotel who had tried so hard to do the right thing, to realize how severe the repercussions can be.

Of course, one way to avoid these problems would be to take the decisions away from everyone. This is what happened in Hitler's Germany. Further, I don't think anyone wants every case involving a doctor and a patient to be decided by a committee somewhere. This would completely immobilize medicine. Thus—who decides in which 1 or 2 per cent of medical cases help will be given to the doctor and/or patient? And then who will provide the crutches to those who need them?

As I said to begin with, the formal decision-making apparatus we need doesn't really function properly at the federal, local, or individual level. We must decide quickly *who shall decide.*

For of all sad words of tongue or pen,
The saddest are these: "It might have been!"
    —JOHN GREENLEAF WHITTIER, *Maud Muller*

�֎

CHAPTER 8

Roadmap for The Unknown*

The foregoing chapters show how difficult it is to determine who in our social fabric should be making some of our critical choices. Thus, it is imperative that we examine carefully any decision-making apparatus, either in use now or about to be introduced, to see what may be involved that bears on the more general question: What should man be like?

I have indicated my recommendations for setting up statutory consultants who are elected and directly responsible to Congress to deal with critical decisions at the federal level. Further, some tentative beginnings have already been made with panels of citizens appointed to handle the local problems of the allocation of time on kidney machines; it is to be hoped that a careful study of their procedures and principles will be undertaken and publicized by some competent individual or group. While these panels are a step in the right direction, their members are being appointed rather than elected. Thus they do not fulfill the important criterion that those forces which must be responsible for a decision should also

*This material is adapted from testimony presented in 1967 to the Judiciary Committee of the Michigan State Senate.

be held accountable. Accordingly, it seems worthwhile to consider a blueprint for a possible apparatus to deal with still another area —abortions—a plan which tries to avoid some of the shortcomings I have been criticizing.

In the past few years, there have been attempts in over half of the fifty states to change the abortion laws. In spite of some fairly violent and well-publicized public discussions, many people still seem to believe that this question can be considered in isolation— that, once either legislation is passed permitting abortion or the whole possibility is rejected the subject will be closed, so to speak. I suspect many of these people have the same moral reservations as I do about abortion, and thus prefer to sweep the whole issue under the rug. Unfortunately, we can't allow this to happen for the abortion dilemma is only the currently visible small fraction of the very large iceberg dealing with the control of quality of human life. Thus, the way we handle or mishandle abortion will probably determine how we handle or mishandle many of the other critical dilemmas (e.g. gene manipulation, spare parts, potent new drugs, mind manipulation) which are just two or three, or five or ten years down the road.

JUST WHEN LIFE BEGINS IS A PROBLEM that presents a stumbling block for many people in making decisions on abortion. Part of the reason there is so much heat generated about this subject is that at least five different points in time are proposed for this critical moment. The conservative Jewish and current Catholic positions are that life begins at conception. There is some disagreement among various adherents to this belief as to whether it means the moment the sperm and egg unite, or when the fertilized egg is actually implanted in the wall of the uterus and begins to divide.

The most common Protestant view today is that life begins at "quickening"—in other words, when the fetus begins to show some movement. In fact, following the precepts of Aristotle and Thomas Aquinas, the Catholic Church in the Middle Ages permitted abortion prior to "fetal quickening."* The Pope in 1588 responded to

---

*It is interesting in this regard that Aristotle believed that quickening began on the fortieth day of pregnancy for a male fetus and on the eightieth day in females; he thought females were misbegotten males.

a variety of pressures by issuing a papal bull forbidding all abortions. This was thoroughly disregarded until 1869, when strong prohibitive action was initiated, and this rule has been Church dogma ever since. Protestant beliefs and practices vary a good deal, but most sects and individuals adhere to the statement issued by the National Council of Churches in 1961: that abortions to save the life or health of the mother or prevent the birth of a grossly malformed child are proper.

Most states give a fetus certain legal rights—equivalent to the recognition of life—at some point. For example, after birth a child may sue for damages it has received as the result of an accident to the mother in the last four or five months of pregnancy. Further, a burial certificate is usually required for a child stillborn after the fifth to seventh month. In some states this whole issue is quite confused, since the moment from which these periods are counted varies. For example, in my state of Michigan, a recent Supreme Court decision stipulates that a child can sue for damages inflicted from the tenth week of pregnancy on. Yet it is not necessary to give a name and a burial prior to the fifth or sixth month.

The liberal Jewish tradition is that life begins just at or prior to birth, and thus there is no prohibition against abortion early in pregnancy. An increasing number of Protestants are also saying that a fetus is not a life until it can be self-sustaining outside the mother. Currently, this would seem to be somewhere along in the sixth month. However, this may fluctuate greatly in the next few years, since we shall probably develop the ability to remove a growing embryo from the mother's womb very early in the pregnancy and continue its uninterrupted growth completely outside the mother in a "test tube." Once such a technique is perfected, it will undoubtedly be widely used to reduce the number of defective births, for many youngsters are born with severe handicaps, not because of genetic defects but because so many things can go wrong in the female reproductive system.

Finally, some groups feel that a child only becomes a human being when it has the important property of self-awareness. Accordingly, in some places a child is given a "birth certificate" or its equivalent only seven to eleven years after birth.

All too often those on the extreme ends of the abortion argument try to hide behind one or the other of the five definitions. Its proponents try to sweep the issue under one rug by defining the beginning of life in such a way that a fetus doesn't qualify for protection, whereas their adversaries make use of a different rug by saying, "A fetus is a life, and we must not take a life." Or repeatedly I hear the statement, "We could stop all this arguing if you scientists would just get busy and get us the facts." Unfortunately, an experiment can never be run which will definitely establish either when life begins or when it ends, because life depends upon what we define it to be. Even though I am a Protestant and adhere to most Protestant views, I believe that life begins when the full potential is there. In other words, once an egg is fertilized and is implanted in the wall of the uterus (or even has been removed to a test tube somewhere) so that it divides and reproduces itself—on a continuing basis—then for me it has fulfilled the primary requisite of life.

On one occasion when I made this statement before a large audience, a man said, "Well, if you believe that a fetus is a life, but advocate abortion, then you are a murderer." Upon further questioning, however, I found that he advocated not giving medical treatment to older people who are in terminal stages of illness. My obvious comment was that I thought he had a rather lopsided definition of murder, since we must face the same fundamental question in dealing with an abortion, euthanasia, capital punishment, or even sending a G.I. into battle. As I see it, we are going to take human lives (e.g., over 40,000 people are killed by autos each year) the only question is, under what circumstances?

We have had numerous state laws to answer this question with respect to abortion. In the earliest abortion law in the United States, passed in Connecticut in 1821, abortion prior to quickening was not an offense; this was the situation in Arkansas and Mississippi as late as 1947 and 1956. Today, 42 states have laws permitting abortion to save the life of the mother, and 6 states have laws allowing an abortion to preserve the health of the mother. The current attempts to change the laws do not introduce something new, but rather change the circumstances in which an abortion can be authorized. In addition, the new laws also make some change in who will decide whether a life shall or shall not be taken.

WHO WILL BE ON THE ABORTION JURIES is, in fact, one of the most important items specified in the new versions of the law. New York in its 1828 law was the first to entrust the medical profession with the decision to abort to save the life of the mother. In current attempts to change the law (all of which derive from a report by a committee of the American Bar Association) the important provisions are as follows: If a district attorney specifies that a woman is pregnant through rape or incest, she can have an abortion; or if three doctors certify that the pregnancy will cause her physical or mental damage, or the child will suffer a gross abnormality, she can have an abortion. This is already the law in Colorado and North Carolina; and in California it is the law, but minus the provision for gross abnormalities. Other states seem almost certain to enact legislation along very similar lines.

A similar attempt was made in Michigan. When I testified before our Senate Judiciary Committee, I stated that although I felt we should enlarge the circumstances in which parents should be allowed to apply for, and secure, authorization for an induced abortion, I felt that the proposed law was a bad one for two reasons.

Most critically, I felt it would not establish appropriate "juries." If in fact it is only a legal question of whether the child has been conceived by rape or incest, then the two-person jury of the district attorney and the mother are appropriate. Or if a fetus is to be treated simply as a tumor or an inflamed appendix, then a jury of four people (three doctors plus the mother) is appropriate to determine the strictly medical questions of whether the mother will suffer physical or mental harm, or the child suffer a gross abnormality. Now, to be sure, there are legal and medical questions involved; nevertheless, since I believe that a *fetus is a life*, I think these are inadequate panels to make such a decision. Certainly once the child is born, so that *everyone* agrees it is a living being, we would not authorize such juries to terminate its life.

Accordingly, I recommended that our Legislature authorize the establishment of regional committees—coinciding with the forty circuit court districts in our state—to decide on parental applications for abortion. To make sure that all the groups and forces which must be considered are represented and held accountable, I proposed that these panels should consist of seven people. There should be an elected representative of the doctors. In addition, there should be an elected representative of the psychiatrists, because if a woman is aborted there is a reasonable chance that she will end up with psychiatric problems in menopause. Not only should one of the four probate judges in a circuit court district represent the legal profession, but the decisions should be processed through his court, since a probate judge normally speaks for those who are not really capable of speaking for themselves. To represent the moral and ethical values in a formal way, I feel that the clergy in that district should elect one of their members. Finally, I urged that there be three members of the public elected at large to look out for the interests and concerns of society. Hopefully, some of these panel members will be women and some men, since there are and should be differing viewpoints on abortions depending upon sex.

In all cases, applications for abortions should be initiated by the parents. Once the applications are received by the elected jury, its deliberations clearly should proceed behind closed doors. An obvious potential disadvantage of such a large committee is that it may act too slowly, since there are only a few weeks after a pregnancy is confirmed during which an abortion can be performed easily and safely. This could be got around, however, by specifying that failure of the committee to *veto* an application within three weeks constitutes authorization of the request. In other words, "pocket approval" rather than pocket veto. Finally, this group should have available very excellent counseling service, so that no matter what the decision is, the parents will receive psychiatric help. Such procedures would probably have insured that the couples I have cited whose lives were shattered by their problems would have had either a needed crutch during their critical period, or help early and throughout their trying time.

So far, I have dwelt on the makeup of the jury. Other features of the proposed legislation must also be considered, however.

The changes proposed in most states are, I feel, good in two respects. First, and most importantly, they increase the number of situations in which abortions can be authorized by adding three critical categories—incest, mental damage to the mother, and gross abnormality of the child—not found in most present regulations. Second, they recognize that rape is so contrary to natural behavior, and the consequences to the mother so great, that the constraints on abortions for pregnancies arising in this way should be removed.

By contrast, most of the proposed legislation seems inadequate in four respects.

1. The "juries" established are not adequate.

2. The father is not involved in the decisions in a formal way. Though in some cases the father may be unknown, while in others it may be better to circumvent him, wherever possible he should participate, since surely a mother does not "own" a child by herself —certainly after birth she does not!

3. It lumps together rape and incest, and also the welfare of the mother, with the welfare of the child. This seems unfortunate, since different principles and rights are involved in making decisions in these categories.

4. Two of the most critical categories—the unwanted child and pregnancies arising in spite of careful contraception—are not considered. This is unfortunate, since many people claim that considerably more than half the illegal abortions now performed involve married women avoiding the birth of an unwanted child.

My evaluation of the virtues and drawbacks of the proposed changes derives from a number of underlying issues. An abortion involves a very complex interplay of the rights of the child-to-be and its parents. The rights of other children in the family and of society in general must be considered also, since a seriously defective child may be involved which requires unusual care or may generate severe family problems. Thus, it is important to consider whose rights are primarily involved in any particular section of the proposed legislative changes, since a different balance is involved in each case.

DO WE REALLY NEED SUCH AN ELABORATE SYSTEM? Obviously the greatest disadvantage of this system is that it again sets up what could be a large bureaucracy. However, on four counts the need is so great that it seems to me we have to pay this price.

First, the number of illegal abortions performed each year is very large: the estimates vary from 100,000 to 1,200,000 (this latter number seems impossibly large, however, since this would mean that one out of four pregnancies is illegally terminated). Most of these are performed by inadequately trained personnel, with the result that 8,000—10,000 women die each year from bungled abortions. Hopefully, these numbers can be drastically reduced by setting up a formal apparatus which will carefully consider applications from parents and will assure that they receive expert and thorough counseling and/or medical care.

Second, as we have seen, there has been a tremendous increase in our ability to predict the chances that a child will have any one of a large number of defects. In particular, our new abilities to predict or make tests about the "quality of life" of the baby-to-be means that we must ask, "Should a child have the right not to be born under conditions of extreme suffering and/or inability to know who and what it is?"

My third reason for advocating this system is that I believe—as has been observed in other countries—that the availability of a formal decision-making apparatus and excellent counseling service will reduce the total number of abortions and drastically reduce those performed by incompetent personnel.

This may not seem consistent with the fact that doctors in Colorado report a sizable increase in requests for legal abortions following passage of their state bill. A similar increase was observed in both Sweden and Japan just after they initiated their abortion programs. However, in both countries there has been a subsequent drop in recent years. Although the reports are not as complete, the same pattern seems to be emerging in Norway. Thus, an important assumption underlying my specific recommendations is that the framework proposed will cause the total number of abortions (legal and illegal) to be reduced. This seems likely not only because the number of applicants may decline, but also because experience indicates that abortion boards will undoubtedly operate in a cautious fashion.

My fourth reason for supporting this kind of system has already been discussed but needs to be repeated. I believe firmly in individual responsibility! Yet there are situations where it is difficult to stand alone—to be an island to ourselves. Abortion is one of these. The consequences can be so great, and occasionally so unpredictable, that parents often need someone to "blame" when a crisis develops. The committees and their staffs should provide an invaluable crutch in this regard to minimize the psychiatric problems that so often arise in the later life of these mothers, and to avoid the build-up of pressures between parents which could disrupt a marriage.

In my own limited experience I have had a few women come to my office "demanding" help to secure an abortion, who really were seeking advice: in fact, many seem eager to have someone talk them out of proceeding, so long as they were given alternative solutions to their problem. Under present restrictions; most women considering abortion seek out first the illegal operator rather than the legitimate doctor, and so the initial and probably decisive advice they receive is not the kind one would like to see them get. If regional committees are given the proper kind of staff, parents should not only get good advice from the start, but would be unlikely to turn to an illegal abortionist if their request were denied. For the proposed committees to exert maximum benefit, their assigned staffs should work carefully to help parents solve their problems, whether their requests are denied or authorized (e.g., through psychiatric counseling, adoption for those who abort a defective child, placement of an unwanted child, and so on).

SOMEONE MUST SPEAK FOR THOSE UNABLE TO SPEAK FOR THEMSELVES. Here is the main reason I have proposed these regional committees with broad representation: one would like to make absolutely certain that someone will speak for the rights of the child, whether it be the right to be born or the right not to be born, depending upon the circumstances! The same voice is needed for the patient in a coma, for the psychiatrically incompetent, or even for someone who may be born into a hopelessly crowded situation where just plain living would be impossible.

The proposed committees have another advantage which is worth reemphasizing. The election of committee members will require the various groups involved to wrestle with the crucial ethical questions concerned. As candidates for committee positions state the criteria they expect to follow in making decisions, the public will affirm their stated values by their vote. This, one may hope, will provide important guidelines for operating in the future, since these other areas deal with the quality of life where we also lack appropriate decision-making groups.

If, in fact, the way we handle or mishandle the abortion issue is likely to set important precedents, then it is crucial that we look carefully at the problems to be encountered in the actual operation of the panels. Accordingly, I propose that the regional committees be authorized initially for only a fixed length of time—perhaps ten years, and that near the end of that period a blue-ribbon panel be given the authority and obligation to go over the records of the regional committees to determine whether the system should be continued, and if so, what changes may be needed. In particular, it is essential that the blue-ribbon panel single out any general operating procedures that may emerge.

WILL YOU PARTICIPATE? This is, of course, the critical question. Recently, changes have already been made in the abortion laws of at least five states, and there will be changes in others before long. Thus decisions are being made right now about *who will decide.*

As indicated above, I do not like certain parts of the new laws, and so am going to do what I can to get my own system adopted. If you don't like the current changes, or my suggestions either, you had better get busy. Above all, don't come back to me ten years from now, damning what I have done and telling me what might have been or should have been. You earn your right to be heard ten years from now by working hard today, tomorrow, this week, this month, this year, when the die is being cast.

In fact, suppose that such an arrangement were set up in your local community and a notice appeared in the newspaper that it was time for candidate petitions to be filed for the three positions to represent the public at large. Would you be willing or even eager to serve as a candidate? In particular, would you be willing to campaign and say, "Here are my beliefs, these are the criteria I will use in deciding whether to approve or veto applications from parents"?

When I asked this question of a group of clergymen, one of the men said, "Before I answer, tell me how many cases such a group would receive." Since the estimates of the number of abortions performed each year vary from 100,000 to 1,200,000, it is impossible to foretell the figure with any great accuracy. However, using what appear to be the most probable estimates, each group would have perhaps approximately 100 applications each year. When the minister got this answer, his immediate reply was, "Let's see, if you lost three nights' sleep over each one, that just about shoots a whole year of sleep."

I know from personal experience that his assessment is not far wrong. Whoever serves on such panels will lose sleep. But the loss will be worth it, if they can begin to provide us with a road map to navigate the unknown.

For it matters not how small the beginning may seem to be:
What is once well done is done forever.
Enter upon your inheritance, accept your responsibilities.
    —WINSTON CHURCHILL, *While England Slept* (1936)

�

CHAPTER 9

The High Cost of Living

The cost of getting involved in some of today's and tomorrow's real-life dilemmas can be very high. When decisions amounting to what I have called "playing God" go wrong, those who are involved invariably get hurt, and badly. Thus, since we have no choice but to play God, there are at least three things which must be done quickly.

I. THESE ISSUES MUST BE DISCUSSED WHILE THERE IS STILL TIME. If we learned one thing from nuclear testing, it is that we dare not wait until the bombs have gone off to begin the discussion. By then people's prejudices are too entrenched and it is extremely difficult to have meaningful dialogue.

Unfortunately, few people in public life are willing to stand up and be counted on most of these issues. This problem is encountered in unexpected ways. Three years ago I was running hard in the Republican primary in Michigan for the United States Senate. During that time I was invited to a small private college to lecture on birth defects; this, of course, makes for a rather unusual campaign speech. Following my convocation talk there was a lot of discussion about questions I had raised, and many other alternatives were considered also.

About a month later a candidate from the opposing party came to the same campus. Needless to say, he did not speak on this topic. Nevertheless, after his formal speech he was asked, "Where do you stand on therapeutic abortion?" I'm told that after his eyes stopped revolving, the student added, "If you don't understand the question, I'll explain it to you," and proceeded to do so at some length. When he had finished the candidate is reported to have said, "Well, I hope it never comes to that."

"You mean you don't want to do anything for these poor unfortunate youngsters?" pressed the student.

After some further thought, the candidate answered, "I guess I'm not prepared to take a stand."

"When will you be?" was the immediate inquiry. At which point came a quiet voice from the back of the room: "The day after election."

Unfortunately, this candidate is not alone. There are few people in public life, whether in the political arena or in the churches and synagogues, who are really willing to speak out on these issues. This is a pity, because the biological bombs I have been describing will have far greater consequences and repercussions than the atomic and hydrogen bombs ever could have. Moreover, these bombs have a very short fuse, and the fuse has been lit. Thus we can no longer afford the luxury of dodging these issues, nor of letting public figures disregard them.

2. once the discussion begins, we dare not let the extremists dominate nor pervert it. Unhappily, this is what happened with nuclear testing. All too often the bombs were claimed to be either all black or all white. Those at one extreme said that they were *the* evil in the world, and if we could just get rid of them somehow everything would be all right. By the same token, the all-white boys said that if we just had enough bombs we could *solve* all the evils of the world. As is now so abundantly evident, neither extreme was correct. But with people arguing from the two extremes, it is very

difficult to find out just what in-between shading of gray is most appropriate. In other words, what is it we want to buy? What are we willing to pay?

It should be evident that the scientific developments I have discussed will be neither all good nor all bad. In each case, we must pay a price to buy some new capability. Thus, once the discussion starts, we dare not let the extremists turn it into a shouting match.

There are other types of extremists of whom we need to beware. One of these is the scientist who may say, "I turned up the knowledge—I dare not entrust the decisions to some of these emotional, nonanalytical humanists." On the other hand, we can't afford the humanist who believes that all scientists are so cold-blooded and inhuman that they can't be trusted. Above all, we cannot let either the scientist or the humanist say that you can't trust the unscrupulous politicians.

All three types of people must cooperate very carefully in bringing their competence to bear, to see that these things get resolved. In many cases, a single person may bring a concern or a competence from more than one of these areas. It is not the label we put on him that is important, but rather what he has to offer and what kind of commitment he is willing to give. Especially we must insist that he not seek for simplistic black-and-white answers which no longer exist.

3. THOSE WHO MUST MAKE THE DECISIONS MUST BE PROPERLY PREPARED. Many, perhaps most of the decisions discussed here will have to be made by the young people in our high schools and colleges today. There are two reasons for this. Let me discuss the more trivial one first.

Much of the science I have been talking about will come to fruition and really be implemented within 25 to 50 years from now. Add 25 years to the ages of those now in our high schools and colleges, and it is their generation that will be in charge of things, whether we or they like it or not. In fact, they may be in charge long before that, unless my generation wakes up and gets moving. This brings me to the second and most important reason why they must be the decisive generation.

I am afraid my generation will not provide the ethical framework within which these decisions must be made. Certainly one recognizes the many hazards of an over-planned society like Hitler's Germany. Even so, we dare not deal with these situations on a day-to-day, catch-as-catch-can basis.

Unfortunately, my contemporaries have overreacted to what was handed on to us by our fathers and grandfathers. In trying to determine what kind of government we should have in the world, they drew up a number of very fine slogans such as "Make the world safe for demoncracy" and so on. But they didn't get the job done, and many of my generation have said "Your absolutes didn't work. There are no absolutes. Everything is relative." This has even slopped over into religion with the arguments from some of the "God is dead" group. Accordingly, mine is now basically a generation of technicians. We will provide the new scientific knowledge, but not the moral framework, I am afraid.

Since our youngsters soon must assume the burdens for these decisions, we had better make sure they are adequately prepared. This means that really we must prepare certain groups within our society quite differently. In any functioning organization, whether it is a school, a church, or a nation, there are invariably four categories of people.

Only about 1 per cent really make the decisions in most organizations. The Communists recognized this early in the game, and in most countries Party members comprise 1 per cent or less of the population.

Secondly, there is a group of 9-10 per cent which I call eager beavers for want of a better term, who agitate to make sure decisions are made: individuals from this group will step up and take over if some of the top decision makers falter.

Once the decisions are made, they must be carried out. Thus about 25 per cent of most groups are technicians.

Finally, the remaining 65 per cent are simply along for the ride. They are not going to participate in a constructive way, no matter what we try to do.

Obviously, the top 10 per cent—the decision makers and the eager beavers—must have a very broad preparation: they must not only know what science is all about, but must also be well versed in the values area. In the future, those who know only science will be equally hazardous for making decisions as those who know no science! Thus we must insist that those unwilling to pay the price of getting this schizophrenic background should stay out of the decision-making role, at least so far as society is concerned.

However, *everyone* really needs to have a more thorough preparation than we are providing today, for though society must set up the apparatus for making decisions, if I have my way most decisions will still be made by only a few people at a time. That is, the family of an individual must have an awful lot to say about questions of euthanasia, and except in cases of incompetence it must be left up to the two people involved as to whether they do or do not procreate a child. Thus, we must provide also a pretty good preparation for the technicians and particularly for the bottom 65 per cent. Although the hangers-on will not participate in a constructive way, they must be aware of the consequences of any action, since the new decisions involve the very nature of man himself. Further, this group must be adequately prepared simply because we dare not take the chance that some rabble-rousers should come along and pervert the decision-making process into a slam-bang argument between those taking extreme positions.

Perhaps you feel uneasy at having the younger generation assume such awesome responsibility so soon. Certainly many have little faith in our current youth. This lack of confidence is not new, of course; Sir Francis Bacon in the early 1600's said, "Young men are fitter to invent than to judge, fitter for execution than for counsel, and fitter for new projects than for settled business."

Yet I don't throw up my hands in horror at our younger generation. Indeed, I am continually impressed by their concern and commitment. My chief worry is whether we may so overwhelm them with "facts" that they lose sight of the importance of value judgments.

WHERE WILL OUR YOUNG PEOPLE GET THE GUIDELINES THEY NEED? One place they will not find them is in science. Science is set up to ask questions such as: How is an atom built? How do our genes control us? How do our minds work? How is the universe constructed?

From these *how* questions we find out what the good Lord has given us to work with. But to put this information to use, we must ask: Why is there an atom? Why does man exist? Why is there a universe at all?

You can't do experiments to investigate these *why's*. Our answers to such questions must come from the belief side of the fence: from religion, philosophy, and the other activities we call the humanities.

Our beliefs and the associated values come from a variety of sources: parents, associates, schools, churches, the news media, and society in general. If any link in this crucial chain fails to function properly, then the individual will probably be in trouble.

As an illustration of how parents can go awry, let me cite a recent situation in which a clergyman friend of mine was consulted. One of his parishioners could not understand how his son had ended up in the penitentiary. His boy had been the lookout while three buddies robbed a filling station and beat the attendant so badly that he almost died. My friend soon discovered that in the past, during Sunday afternoon drives in the family station wagon, the son had been posted in the seat facing to the rear, his assignment being to keep an eye out for the police as his father whizzed along at ten to fifteen miles per hour above the speed limit. Another young man in less trouble summed up both situations when he said, "I guess I never could hear what my Dad was saying about values because his cheating on Mother and on his income-tax returns shouted so loud."

Often in the teaching profession we also allow our actions to speak louder than our words. Most educators try to get across to students that it is important to have integrity, responsibility, and concern for our fellows. However, the lessons begin to fall on deaf ears when a school like Columbia University allows 300 student rebels and another 300 people from off campus to prevent 27,000 legitimate students from getting their proper education. In this case, fundamental values and rights were disregarded by *both* students (who employed fascist-type techniques) and administrators (who obviously had little rapport with the faculty and showed inadequate regard for the rights of *all* the students).

Public officials can also provide a negative example in a variety of ways. If rioting and looting are tolerated in some situations, then there will almost certainly be an increase in other forms of violence throughout society. Moreover, we cannot tolerate discrimination on the basis of race or creed or color in jobs, housing, or education and then expect those who are discriminated against—or even, in fact, those who discriminate—to obey the rest of the rules of society.

Finally, civil rights illustrates how we committed church people have fallen down badly. We preach the universal brotherhood of man, and yet the most segregated hour of the week is 11:00 A.M. Sunday morning. Can we allow this to continue and then really expect our youngsters to understand when we try to teach them the Golden Rule?

In spite of the occasional failure of some of us as parents, educators, public officials, or just plain citizens, this is an impressive generation coming up. I have great respect for what they have already accomplished as a group. As one person said, "They are hypercritical but not hypocritical."

Hypercritical they should be, for all too often we oldsters live one set of values and preach another. One of my own main concerns is whether they themselves can avoid hypocrisy. Although they cry out for everyman's rights, a few of the activists claim their cause is so holy that they can go into the streets and usurp the rights of others; although they proclaim that everyone must love his fellow man above all else, many strive for selfish gratification in free love or LSD trips which impose a severe, lifelong price on another human being; although they decry hypocrisy, a few of the radicals claim that an honest and democratic society can only be achieved by anarchy in the streets of Chicago and elsewhere.

Whether they can escape from their own hypocrisy depends upon the new leadership they so desperately need. So far, their protests have been mainly negative. Even so, they have rendered valuable service by calling attention to important defects in our society. New leadership is now needed to undertake the positive job of correcting these deficiencies. If it is not developed quickly, then they will be just as hypocritical as those they now criticize. God help us all if the control of human heredity, or the use of mind manipulation, or the allocation of spare parts, are decided in the streets.

WHERE WILL SOCIETY FIND ITS VALUES? is thus the crucial question. Fortunately many of the needed fundamental beliefs are already "built in." For example, people in the communications industry state flatly that the public should never be allowed to make decisions based almost exclusively upon facts, but that they should always be entrusted with those that deal primarily with values. Very often, indeed, the public gets ahead of its "leaders" in formulating value judgments.

In this day of the mass-advertising dictum that there is a sucker born every second, and that we are all shallow and easily manipulated, it is seriously tempting to downgrade the American public. In fact, I must admit that when I first began to receive a large number of requests to speak on the ethical problems arising from science, my colleagues and I were dubious that the general public would be interested or would listen. In essence, I began my series of lectures pessimistically, but with the conviction that one way to make sure the American public did not listen and did not address itself to these problems would be *not* to give them any exposure. Fortunately, I have been continually and pleasantly surprised by all types of groups, and my assessment of the good common sense and dedication of the public in general has gone up tremendously. When you approach an audience on the basis of expecting them to be responsible and concerned, they will be.

A significant point is that even before I give a talk I know what the questions will be, since the same twenty or twenty-five general questions are asked independent of the groups involved. The only difference is that a junior high school youngster begins in a halting way, and when he is about halfway through says, "Oh well, you know what I mean." By contrast, one of my colleagues usually prefaces his inquiry by a long statement, a number of qualifications, and then finally comes to the question mark.

Occasionally, I find an audience which refuses at first to come to grips with these questions, apparently for the same reason I have sometimes avoided an issue until a case comes up where an answer must be given. All too often my rational processes come smack into conflict with one or more of my deep-seated prejudices. When this happens, I want time to reexamine very carefully that initial gut reaction, for I have learned from sad experience that all too often

I can't trust my prejudices. Yet, by the same token, I realize more and more that there is no set way of arriving at a completely rational decision on questions which must rest on fundamental beliefs about the nature of life, the nature of man's identity and existence, and similar considerations. And when reason and beliefs come into conflict, which should we trust?

Needless to say, I have done a lot of hard thinking about which of my old beliefs are still valid and which must be revised. Happily, much of the public is doing the same today: this reassessment is perhaps most evident publicly among Catholics.

The search for values is particularly crucial because the sources of our ethics have changed greatly in recent years. In the past our values came principally from either the churches or the matriarchs. The church was not only the place of worship but also the central meeting place in small communities. As a consequence, it had a profound influence on all types of citizens. But we are no longer a collection of small towns, and the churches are seeking hard today to find their proper role.

Further, before achieving "equality," women held an exalted position. Thus, in many communities the moral code was drawn up and administered by the Tuesday afternoon bridge club, or the Wednesday sewing circle, or the Friday morning Bible study group, and so on. As I know from personal experience, the administration of the code could be pretty brutal, but the framework was there and readily recognizable. All too often today that is not the case; as a girl said in one of my classes, "My mother is nothing but a social chairman and taxi driver." Accordingly, where do we turn?

I hope both groups come into their own again soon. Perhaps you disagree—perhaps you don't like either the churches or the matriarchs. If not, you had better find—quickly—a source of values that is satisfactory to you. Interrelated as our society is today, we shall all profit or suffer from the way you perform as you encounter these dilemmas. As Longfellow said in "The Poets,"

> Not in the clamor of the crowded street,
> Not in the shouts and plaudits of the throng,
> But in ourselves, are triumph and defeat.

As I know from the few counseling cases in which I have had some part, the moment of decision involving a life is indeed a lonely one. At that crucial time, no matter how much counseling help may be available, no matter how many prayers are said, finally an individual must face himself and rely on his own inner resources to find "triumph or defeat." Once made, the decision and its consequences must then be lived with forever. The necessary maturity to make and live with tough decisions is possessed only by those who have a solid set of personal values.

In the current uncertainty and searching, one hears repeatedly one particular question: Will we get our values from religion, or will we have a rational system? Clearly such a questioner knows little about how an ethical system is constructed. Any worthwhile system must be based upon a set of fundamental premises. From this base, a set of operating procedures can then be rationalized. The only question is where we get the basic premises—by divine revelation, from the Scriptures, from the contemplation of some new prophet, by observing what has worked down through history, by some supposed reasoning process, or out of thin air? But since we are here for only a brief period and thus can never experience eternal truth personally, these basic *premises* must be precisely that —statements (or assumptions) about what we believe to be true today.

I HAVE FOUND FIVE FUNDAMENTAL BELIEFS UPON WHICH I MUST RELY AS I WRESTLE WITH VARIOUS CASES. These are the things about which one must take a stand with oneself while trying to arrive at a decision about what to do. To choose a particular course of action in a given situation I must assign some particular importance, or weight, to each of these values.

1. *There is a basic orderliness in the way things interact throughout our universe.* Wherever I look I find orderliness—whether it be in the atom, our genes, our minds (at least the male mind), or the universe in general. On the basis of these observations, I *believe* that there should also be an orderliness in the way we humans treat each other. Of course, this implies that there is right and wrong, and so in this sense I differ from many who argue that everything is completely relative.

Actually, even many of the operating principles of two thousand years ago are still valid today. Nevertheless, a goodly number of today's situations are so new that much of the old dogma is inadequate. In some of the cases I have encountered I have had to ask myself whether I must seek some new form of order in human relations or consider merely some reinterpretation or extension of an old operating procedure. Without exception I find that the centuries-old *fundamental* values are still vital and adequate. But it is very evident that, with circumstances becoming so complex and so varied, we can no longer *codify* the actual *operating* procedures to be used in each and every situation, as was done in the past. Instead of restrictive laws the lawyers and politicians must establish proper decision-making units within which our citizens can operate. And instead of dogmatic operating rules, our theologians and others in the humanities need to make sure that people have sound and orderly fundamentals, so that they can operate from commitment and compassion in the wide variety of situations now arising.

2. *This orderliness was established by a concerned creator.* Often people do not realize that science and religion have one thing in common. As a scientist I must believe that there is this orderliness, otherwise there is no sense in my doing experiments to discover its outlines. Similarly it is necessary to believe in orderliness in order to worship its creator.

The only question really is, was the order created or did it arise by itself? I happen to believe very strongly that it was created by God.

As an experimental scientist I really don't need to worry about this question as I go about my day-to-day business. However, in deciding whether a child should or should not be aborted, it makes quite a big difference that I do believe a fetus is a life endowed by a creator.

3. *Life has a sanctity which should not be casually violated.* This book reflects my profound respect and concern for the sanctity of life. Yet my whole concept of "life" has changed quite dramatically in the last few years. In the past I knew quite clearly what life was: a person was either alive or dead and there wasn't much in between. Because of the more recent advances described here, we must now be concerned with the *quality* of life. Further, we must be con-

cerned with various facets of life. Specifically, we must take into account not only the sanctity of biological life, but also the sanctity of psychological life. In many cases our concern in these three areas may come into direct conflict. For example, in the case of the family having a third mongoloid child, I felt we would be violating one aspect of the sanctity of the child's life if it were terminated by an abortion; yet undoubtedly we would also be violating its future psychological and social well-being if it were not aborted. And certainly the psychology of the parents and the doctor would be affected in quite different ways by an abortion.

Faced with this increasing complexity, many people still hold to the naïve view that morality is really nothing more than a question of premarital sex or no premarital sex. One *only partially* hypothetical situation may illustrate how outmoded that oversimplified approach is today.

Suppose one Saturday night three couples in neighboring motel rooms each procreate a life. The first couple is not married, and when they separate the next morning never see each other again. Further, the mother insists upon keeping the child with her in a small town, and it is socially ostracized. The couple in the next room are married all right, but they have defective genes, and know it, and still go ahead and procreate a child which spends most of its days in suffering in an institution, not knowing who or what it is. The third couple is kosher all the way: they are married, they have good genes, but unfortunately they do not give the child a proper set of values, and so he ends up in a penitentiary.

Which couple is the most immoral?

Some might argue that this question is impossible to answer because everything is relative. Actually, the question is impossible to answer precisely because there *are* absolutes, and the three situations were chosen deliberately to depend solely on a single absolute. Clearly, the sanctity of the first child's social life was violated by subjecting it to ostracism; the second couple disregarded the biological rights of their child by saddling it with a set of defective genes and consigning it to a lifetime of suffering; while the last couple neglected the psychological well-being of their child.

Although I am usually most concerned with the social well-being of *individuals*, we dare not disregard the well-being of society itself.

Society is itself an organism, and we must be every bit as concerned about the sanctity of its life as for that of any inividual man or woman. If we are not, then there will be insufficient orderliness to protect the biological and psychological well-being of individuals, in turn.

4. *There is a "hereafter."* Whenever I am concerned with decisions involving spare parts and/or euthanasia in particular, an important consideration must be whether there is or is not something after our life here on earth. I cannot imagine that we would have been given such sophisticated brains only to deal with our existence here on earth. Thus, I believe there will be a participation by my soul or my spirit—I don't know what form it will take—in a greater scheme of things.

5. *Agape must be the most important principle governing the behavior of people toward people.* The concept that there is a nonpassionate, nonselfish concern which should direct our love for our fellow men is probably the most significant thing enunciated by Christ and other religious leaders. Whenever I am tempted to say no to someone seeking my help, I must always pause and ask once again, "What does it mean to be my brother's keeper?" For me, agape implies that I have a very strong obligation not to walk by on the other side of the road and disregard the fellow human who is "lying in the ditch" needing help.

There are undoubtedly those who would say I shouldn't have stuck my nose into the business of the couple who were fearful of having a third mongoloid child. Perhaps. But I felt, when they asked me for help, that to be a good Samaritan meant I had to lose some sleep and perhaps suffer some psychological scars, to at least try to help them.

It is perhaps important to note that I have not listed honesty as one of the fundamental values, even though I abhor fibbing to cover up personal shortcomings or oversights, whether it be someone else or myself who yields to the temptation. However, a big fat lie to protect someone else's well-being in some cases may be the right thing to do. In fact, it may be the only way to really be my brother's or sister's keeper in some situations.

Perhaps you are every bit as uncomfortable as I have been, and still am, at having to face up to these new responsibilities. Fortunately, most of us are humble enough not to make decisions of this magnitude very casually. But because of the new scientific developments things have changed.

WE NEED A REORIENTATION OF MAN'S ROLE. Throughout recorded history there have been quite large fluctuations in man's concept of his role and responsibility. In earliest times we had a god of fire, a god of the hunt, a god of war, a god of love, and so forth. Since man was completely at the mercy of the gods, it was felt that we could do little or nothing for ourselves. This attitude slowly changed, so that by Old Testament times the Jews had the concept of a covenant between God and man, in which the overall relationship was that of a general and his first lieutenants. Christ set man's status and responsibilities at a maximum: in his teachings we are treated as a part of God. Ever since, there has been a continual decline in the view of man's relative stature. But now, with our new capabilities and obligations, we must reconsider very carefully our self-concepts and our notions of what our role should be. In this connection it is perhaps worthwhile to look once again at those surprisingly few people who have been primarily responsible for the major changes in our concepts of ourselves.

Aristotle and Plato played key parts in the development of the early idea of the duality of man. Basically they formalized the concept, which had grown up apparently in ancient Persia, that body and spirit are distinctly different aspects of man and contribute to quite different desires and goals.

The Jews advanced the status of man significantly with their idea that not only is there only one God, but further, he expects man to act in copartnership with him. In fact, they viewed the relationship as one in which the contractual obligations should be spelled out in a covenant.

Building on this idea of our stature and standing, Christ—particularly as interpreted by Paul to the Greek and Roman world—brought man to his highest state of dignity and also to his greatest sense of need and obligation. Jesus spoke of a oneness with God and of a much more intimate rapport than Jewish tradition envisaged, in which the elation was essentially that of father and son. While he spoke of the need for humility, he also stressed the obligation for involvement and not walking by on the other side of the road when our brother needs help.

Following Christ the changes in our concept of ourselves have almost invariably represented a downgrading of our overall role and identity. St. Augustine and Thomas Aquinas reemphasized the Persian and Greek concepts of the duality of man. In particular, they focused on the notion that the body is evil, while the spirit is good. This was further underlined by both Luther and Calvin, and served as an important basis for Luther's emphasis on the dictum "Ye are saved by faith alone." Kant and Descartes, on the contrary, both emphasized the supremacy of man and the need for rational analysis. In this regard Luther was somewhat schizophrenic, not only in his behavior but also in his preachments: while he talked about the need for relying totally on faith and throwing ourselves on the mercy of a completely overwhelming God, he likewise emphasized the priesthood of all believers—i.e., the obligation of individual responsibility.

Important findings in science also contributed significantly to the general downgrading of man's stature and dignity. When Copernicus presented his evidence that the earth is not only not the center of the universe, but rather a second-rate planet going around a third-rate sun, off on one edge of a medium-sized galaxy, people at first argued that this must be false; then later, when the findings were accepted, the conclusion was that man is far less significant than initially thought. Darwin's theory of evolution had equally earth-shaking impact on many people's ideas about our status. Certainly the continuing evidence that probably life has evolved over many millions of years on this earth, and further, that there is probably life on numerous other planets, again has caused many people either to rebel and refuse to accept the evidence, or else to feel painfully that man is nothing. Unfortunately, it has not occurred to a good many of them that, if we are not as unique as we once thought, we should not so much downgrade man as upgrade God in terms of the complexity and sophistication of this whole creation.

Freud's theories also have contributed to the general idea that man has limited capabilities. In particular, his concept of the *id* as that part of the mind over which we have no real control, plus his sex theories, led to the idea that we are pretty much at the mercies of our own drives and subconscious. Karl Marx's idea of economic determinism also seemed to say that man is subject to forces over which the individual has little or no control.

Einstein's findings have provided an important pressure in the other direction, however. His demonstration that prediction could lead to tremendous control of our physical environment has reestablished man as a decisive and controlling force in the universe once again. Important as the control of our physical environment has been and can be, still the important discoveries in this century will be those in the biological and psychological areas. Not because the physical scientists are going to lie down on the job, but rather because of the fantastic implications of our new outlook in biology.

With important discoveries in the past, man was forced to ask again the questions of *What is man?* and *Why is he here?* Unfortunately, many of these reassessments led to century-long controversies. Now, reassessment is necessary once more, for the biological scientists are giving reason to ask, not only what man is, but the further question of what would we like him to be—and then are giving us the power to do something about it! Undoubtedly we will have controversy once again, as we establish a new set of covenantal relationships to deal with our upgraded status and responsibilities.

In reassessing our role, we must strike a delicate balance between a number of conflicting attitudes. For example, we dare not be overwhelmed by the complexity of the problems which we face and must resolve. What I especially see are the fantastic opportunities now being presented by our new capabilities. But we never get something for nothing. Invariably, whenever the opportunity is great, the price for failure is equally large. Thus it is today.

To illustrate: my only brother is a mongoloid. I don't think anyone can comprehend how much I would give to be able to go in and short-circuit the extra chromosome in each of his cells. That is the sort of opportunity we are talking about. But if we are overwhelmed by the problems, we will be immobilized. By the same token, we dare not disregard them, for if we pay no attention they will only get bigger. Thus, we must face our problems head on, and do our best to resolve them, so that as the opportunities come along we can buy the most and pay the least.

Yet we dare not ever become arrogant or callous, for even though we have no choice but to play a superhuman kind of role, we can never *be* God. That is, being finite, we must always proceed on the basis of incomplete knowledge, hypotheses, and beliefs. However, the fact that we do not have total knowledge does not release us from the obligation, nowadays, to make decisions which we formerly left to God. This is what I meant when I chose the title for this book.

"Too little and too late"—these are bitter words. If you feel the same sense of urgency as I, but are still reluctant to get involved directly, then I would like to paraphrase for you another famous observation: All that is necessary for evil to triumph is that good men and women do nothing *in time*.

The time is very short. We had better get busy—*today!*

When I was a child I spake as a child, I understood as a child, I thought as a child, but when I became a man I put away childish things.

I Corinthians 13:11

✖

CHAPTER 10

The Days of Our Adolescence

One morning soon after he was a year old, my son Davey suddenly said, "Daddy—what's that?" To an already proud papa, this was final proof that we have a little genius. Even disregarding fatherly pride, however, Davey's first recognizable words were quite symbolic, because they and his subsequent phrases and actions parallel all of mankind's historical development. It seems worthwhile to dwell briefly on this parallelism, since this book is about mankind's "coming of age."

When Davey first arrived in this world, my wife and I of necessity had to be his gods: we had to control his destiny completely since our little "blob" could do nothing for himself. But quickly he began to observe and explore, so that his first words expressed his curiosity to one of his creators. And that inquiry has never ceased as he seeks continually to find the rules by which his environment is organized. Even with limited knowledge he has moved rapidly to establish control over at least parts of his actions. By twenty-two months he began to ask for specific items, and at twenty-three months he gave his first orders for action—in fact, by two years he was remarkably adept at manipulating our home, and Grandma posed no hurdle whatsoever from the beginning. As he learns more of the rules, he must of necessity become an adult. That is, he must not only control his own life, but must participate in so far as he is capable in governing his fellow men.

So it is with mankind! Until only recently man has been almost completely at the mercy of the fates, or the gods, or God, since we could do almost nothing about controlling the really important parts of our destiny. For example, it has taken hundreds of years for even a fraction of mankind to wrest political control away from the very few and take this responsibility into their own hands. In the last 50 years, we have been able to determine enough of the rules by which our universe works so that we can control at least parts of our environment here on earth. Now, suddenly, in the last 25 years we have begun to acquire enough knowledge to control the very essence of man himself. Once we learn enough of the rules, like Davey we must assume adulthood by determining the very nature, and thus ultimately the future course, of all mankind.

Clearly, the advances discussed throughout this book provide tremendous opportunities, but also pose fantastic dilemmas of how to put this new information to proper use. The basic scientific knowledge is neither good nor bad; it simply tells us the rules by which our universe operates. But although scientific discovery is amoral, a tremendous amount of good or evil can ensue when we put these things to use.

Perhaps even now you throw up your hands in horror and argue that man should never be so arrogant as to "play God." Nonsense! Each of us is here today because two people played God—they procreated a life. The only real question is how deliberate we should be in determining the quality of that life. Elizabeth and I will do everything within our power to give Davey and his little sister Kim every piece of information and every tool they need to become adults. God has done the same for mankind—he has given us sophisticated brains and has let us find the rules by which much of our universe operates. I cannot believe we would have these wonderful minds if we were only meant to dance at the end of a string like marionettes acting out a prearranged script.

Once these tools become available, no matter what we do—whether we choose to use these techniques or deliberately do not use them, or even attempt to hide our heads in the sand and disregard the alternatives—we shall be making Godlike decisions. The question is not whether we will or will not play God, but whether we have it in us to do it in the responsible way adults should, or in the trivial, irresponsible way of the child who does not face up to the task of determining his own destiny.

Even if we do face our responsibilities, there are again two ways we can proceed which parallel Davey's options. When he grows up he can go off completely on his own, in effect saying, "Dad is no longer relevant and has nothing to offer me." Alternatively, he may decide I did know what I was talking about during his infancy and adolescence, and choose to walk hand in hand with me as an adult.

Mankind faces the same choice. We may decide that since now we are acquiring the capability of literally controlling our own nature and destiny, we no longer need God. Like Davey, we too can go off on our own arrogant way. But I hope not! Just as I look forward to Davey and Kim checking back occasionally with Elizabeth and me, I trust mankind will walk hand in hand with the source of our being and values, once we have achieved adulthood.

The time of decision is upon us! For almost all of history, man has been in his infancy because we could not control our destiny. But with our current explosion of knowledge we are now in the midst of 25 (or at most 100) years of puberty and adolescence. It appears almost certain that the first generation which will have the knowledge, and thus must assume these fantastic new responsibilities, is in our high schools and colleges right now. They are the *first generation of adulthood for all mankind*, for they must make the vital decisions.

Although they may be the *decisive* generation, those of us who are older are the *critical* generation, since we must make sure that they have (*a*) a functioning decision-making apparatus, (*b*) the facts about what is possible, and above all (*c*) help in finding the necessary ethical framework within which to make the needed choices. In essence, it is 11:59 P.M., and before midnight we must provide our Cinderellas and Prince Charmings with a sturdy coach and trustworthy road map to find their way, or else all our dreams and hopes will indeed become rotting pumpkins.

Thus let me end as I began, with the admonition: Come, let us work together humbly, prayerfully, and above all responsibly as we proceed in this awesome business. For the success or failure with which we "play God" in the next few years will determine whether these are the first few moments in mankind's greatest and most exciting hour or the last few seconds in his ultimate tragedy.

✖

A COMPILATION OF CRITICAL QUESTIONS FOR DISCUSSION

(The numbers in parentheses indicate the approximate percentages of people who usually vote YES, NO, and UNDECIDED on each question. I would appreciate it if you would send me a postcard indicating how you vote on these questions.)

1. Should a 66-year-old surgeon who serves about 500,000 people in a remote area accept a kidney transplant from his 22-year-old grandson who is married, has a child two years old and another on the way and who is a promising graduate student in medical research? (10, 65, 25)
2. Suppose after the kidney transplant, the grandson's other kidney goes bad while grandad is still alive, should the kidney be returned to the grandson? (5, 10, 85)
3. If your first child died of amaurotic idiocy so that with one chance in four any children you and your spouse procreated would die from convulsions and seizures, and further if during a pregnancy amniotic fluid had been removed and you found that twice as many of the fetal cells had abnormal fatty deposits as your own blood cells, would you want an abortion? (45, 20, 35)
4. If you were on an abortion jury, would you vote to abort a fetus you knew was going to be microcephalic? (75, 15, 10)
5. If you were on an abortion panel, would you vote to abort a fetus you knew was going to have PKU? (20, 40, 40)
6. Would you be willing to file as a candidate for an abortion jury and then in the campaign to state your beliefs and the criteria you would use in making decisions on applications for abortions? (15, 40, 45)
7. If you have a seriously defective recessive gene (e.g., for muscular dystrophy, cystic fibrosis, or amaurotic idiocy), would you want to take the chance of being injected with a virus which had been shown to correct a comparable defective gene in animals? (50, 35, 15)
8. If we could really develop the capability of gene manipulation, would you want to specify everything about the genetic makeup of your child prior to conception? (5, 70, 25)

9. Would you deliberately choose to have a child with an I.Q. of 200? (10, 50, 40)

10. Do you really want to know what your chances are for procreating a defective child? (40, 40, 20)

11. If you knew your chances of having a seriously defective child were 1 out of 4, would you get married? (50, 25, 25)

12. If you knew your chances were 1 out of 4 of having a child who would not know who and what it is, would you procreate any children? (20, 60, 20)

13. Which of the following three do you advocate:
    a. Continuing our present medical practice which keeps many people alive long enough to pass on their defective genes and thus causes more defective children to be born? (10)   or
    b. Stopping the medical practice for a selected group of people so as to halt the continual pollution of the genetic pool? (5)   or
    c. Embarking upon the road of genetic manipulation with all the hazards involved? (85)

14. Should we as a society deliberately try to "improve man"? (40, 25, 35)

15. Should a decision as to whether to have or not to have a defective child be left strictly up to the parents (even those with I.Q.'s of 35 or 50) (25, 50, 25)

16. If two parents beat a child so that they cripple it for life, should the child be taken away from them? (100, 0, 0)

17. If two parents will have a crippled child, should they be prevented from having children? (65, 20, 15)

18. If the chance that two parents will have a crippled child is 1 out of 4, should they be prevented from having children? (15, 65, 20)

19. Should some children have the right never to be conceived at all if they will not know who and what they are and know only a life of suffering? (65, 25, 10)

20. If the victim of an automobile accident has a heart and lungs which can be kept operating by an appropriate machine, but a brain which will never again operate, and a patient in the hospital desperately needs a heart transplant, would you vote to turn off the sustaining machine and let the heart and lung stop operating "naturally"? (90, 5, 5)

21. Suppose all the conditions above were the same except that there was one in the hospital who needed a heart transplant, would you still vote to turn off the machine? (70, 10, 20)

22. Would you be willing to serve on the trial jury where a man was beaten so badly that he had no electrical activity in the brain, but his heart was removed and put into a man where it beat for another week, and there is a charge of manslaughter against those who had beaten him up? (15, 50, 35)

23. Do you want to have the legal right to choose your time of dying? (60, 25, 15)

24. Should we able to make carbon copies (identical twins except in terms of age) of ourselves and store them away as a complete supply of spare parts for ourselves? (5, 75, 20)

25. Is a person's identity completely determined by his brain?   (10, 70, 20)

26. Would you plug in a respirator for a newborn microcephalic child if you knew that it would be blind, deaf, and have epileptic seizures if it survived? (20, 60, 20)

27. Would you plug in a respirator for a five-year-old microcephalic child who weighed only 17 pounds because it screams all of the time? (30, 40, 30)

28. Would you plug in a respirator for a child with amaurotic idiocy who was having periodic seizures and convulsions? (30, 30, 40)

29. Would you plug in a respirator for an infant with PKU, knowing that if he survived, he must remain on the rigid diet and still will suffer appreciable reduction in his I.Q. from what it would be normally, and further, probably his children will also suffer some intelligence deficit? (40, 30, 30)

30. If your 89-year-old grandmother who has degenerated quite badly in both body and mind in the past few years went into a coma, would you ask a doctor to make her comfortable for only a few days rather than keeping her alive for weeks or perhaps even months if possible? (95, 5)

31. Should the immediate family be the ones to decide whether a person in a terminal illness should or should not be treated even if there is a fairly large inheritance involved? (50, 10, 40)

32. After we decide that the population cannot increase further, should a grandparent get a new kidney or heart if his or her staying alive means that the grandchildren cannot get a permit to have children? (10, 15, 75)

33. If we begin to negotiate treaties concerning levels of populations, should we negotiate only if all countries participate? (80, 10, 10)

34. Should the U. S. provide foreign aid only to those countries which have effective population control programs underway? (60, 25, 15)

35. Should the U. S. require that those countries which receive food from us set aside at least 25% of the value of this food in their own currency for the training of their nationals to be joint agricultural experts and population control experts? (65, 15, 20)

36. Should we develop a new product which can be inserted uner the skin of any woman to give her essentially 100% contraception so long as she desires it? (60, 20, 20)

37. Should we use mind manipulation techniques to change the basic values of criminals? (70, 20, 10)

38. Should we use "cattle prods" to correct seriously abnormal behavior? (75, 15, 10)

39. Should parents in general be responsible for the values in their children? (75, 25)

40. Should parents use either mind manipulation or behavior manipulation techniques to make sure what values are in their children? (10, 50, 40)

41. Should we deliberately impose values on the ghetto child in an attempt to get him "up and out"? (50, 30, 20)

42. Of the following, who should decide whether a drug is or is not tested in a human:
    a. The Food and Drug Administration? (20)

   b. The doctor involved? (20)
   c. The individual (or his parents)? (30) (Undecided: 30)
43. Should only the individual parents be the ones to decide what gene manipulation will be performed in them so as to affect their children? (40, 40, 20)
44. Of the final three applicants to get onto the kidney machine, would you have chosen the 62-year-old author? (25) or the 55-year old alcoholic mother of three? (1-2) or the 37-year-old father of three children who was very active in his community but had deserted his family? (30) (Undecided: 45)
45. Do you think that a doctor should provide a "crutch" to his patients by making their decisions for them? (45, 35, 20)
46. Do you think society should provide a "crutch" to some people by making their decisions for them? (35, 55, 10)